Verity Writes Again

Verity Writes Again

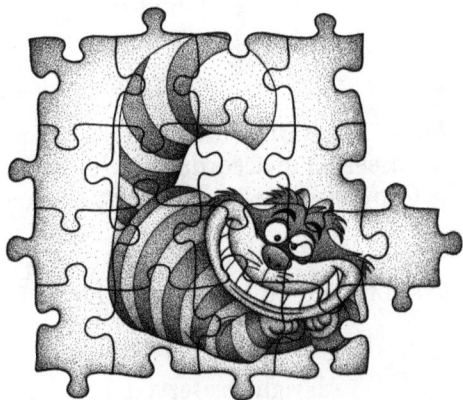

Maria Mann

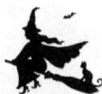

easyBroom

Verity Writes Again

An easyBroom book

Copyright © 2015 Maria Mann

ISBN 978-0957628816

The right of Maria Mann to be identified as the author of this work has been asserted in accordance with Sections 77 and 78 of the Copyright, Designs and Patents Act 1988

Illustrations and Cover Design: Maria Mann

A catalogue record of this book is available from The British Library

Maria Mann is the author of the best selling

Verity Red's Diary
A story of surviving M.E.

&

Love & Best Witches

She has had M.E. for twenty two years, and when she
is not working on her books, loves to curl-up
under blanket of warm cats.

for Seka Nikolic, Auntie Jeanette and Uncle Keith

&

*In memory of Uncle Joe, Julian and
little Mary Poppins*

Acknowledgements

A whole book full of thank yous to my partner Nigel and his brother Jess, for their wonderful help and advice, making it possible and a pleasure, to publish this book myself. Cheers also to Emma, for printing out a nice big template to help me design the cover, and Steve for his wise words regarding printing in the digital age.

Many thanks also to Louise for her sweet verse and drawings; Kira, Len and Jim, for their delightful poetry, and everyone who sent me lovely text messages.

Last but not least to Purrdita, Cleopatra and Tinkerbell; for their inspiration, warm furry love, and marvellous muddy paw prints all over my manuscript.

Prologue

Verity Red (veri tyred) is back, with her mischievously wry wit and bad hair days. She still loves a chocolate treat, watching *Coronation Street*, collecting stray cats that appear on her doorstep, and Christmas gift catalogues that appear on her doormat. Her new *love* is sending text messages from her mobile phone, and she is going to learn to *love* jigsaw puzzles.

Verity's diary begins on 1st September, because in previous months, all her precious energy has gone into writing a book *(Love & Best Witches)* and getting it published. The proof copy is about to arrive, but she's not sure it's such a good idea any more. Somebody might actually read it, after they've briefly flicked through, glancing at the illustrations. What will they think of it? Will anyone want to read a book about a witch who has M.E.?

Christmas gift catalogues have started to arrive with the post, and she is looking forward to curling-up under a blanket of warm cats, while her fingers do the walking.

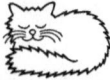

Chapter
One

September

Wednesday 1ˢᵗ

I've done it! I've done it!! *Yes!! Yes!! Yesssssss!!!!!!!!!!* I've survived eight months of another year. Only four months to go and I'll have survived the year 2010. Ten out of ten! Full marks for me! *Another year* of coping with M.E. And myself. *And* I'm still alive. And I'm still sane. Well, most days.

I deserve a HUGE certificate with a fancy border, as big as my bedroom wall. No, bigger! Tall and wide as the billboards in town. Tall and magnificent as the sycamore trees at the end of my garden.

Tall as a tree..... I've survived M.E...... Wonderful, wonderful, *marvellous* me. I feel a poem coming on..... yes... yes... *yes!*

No. Maybe not today.

Thursday 2ⁿᵈ

Dear diary, I'm so sorry I've neglected you this year, until now. You see, all my energy, my spare precious energy, has gone into writing and illustrating a book, for people with M.E. *And* I published it myself! With the help of Ben and his family of course. It's taken five long years, but it's finally completed. The proof copy is due to arrive soon. Very soon.

I've *finally, finally,* done it. Even though my brain is foggy, muddled and dyslexic most of the time; my memory and concentration so poor, I've had few mental pennies to spend, and I've had to re-write everything countless times before it's legible enough for Ben to type.

My right arm dropped off, but an osteopath screwed it back on again; my neck turned into a block of concrete, crumbled, and my head fell off. Another osteopath screwed that back on again too. Then my eyeballs fell out and rolled all over the carpet, so I washed the cat hairs off them under the cold tap, and a kind optician popped them back into their sockets.

But the book is finally done. Completely completed. *At last, at last. HURRAH!*

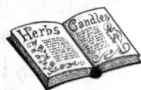

1

Friday 3rd

Oh God. I've actually written a book. One hundred and fifty three whole pages. Will *anyone* buy it?

I need to promote it. I'm not well enough to travel about doing book signings, but many people who have M.E. are housebound anyway. Those well enough to attend a book signing would find standing in a queue exhausting. Well, I'd like to imagine there would be a queue. More than three people would be quite nice.

I had a dream last night, that I was sitting at a table in the book section of WH Smith, signing copies of my book. There was a long queue, through the shop and down the high street, past The Body Shop and Mothercare, M&S and McDonalds. Some people were in wheelchairs. Several crawled on their hands and knees. A witch flew around on her broomstick, cackling wildly. There were a few bats and owls flying around too. This made a young girl in a wheelchair giggle, and a man crawling on his hands and knees, fell over laughing.

Spooky Gothic music filled the air, entertaining everyone, because queuing can be *so boring*, and *so tiring*. If you are in a queue in town, you can do a bit of people watching, but the thrill of that soon wears off, and you desperately feel the need to move two or three steps, *and* you wish you were in a game of Monopoly, so you could throw a double six and move twelve paces forward.

Characters from The Munsters strolled by, singing *The Monster Mash*. They handed out treats to everyone; pumpkin fairy cakes, bat buns, chocolate frogs and rainbow jelly snails (with horns and tails). There was magical pumpkin juice in small plastic cups, because it's not a good idea to drink a lot when you are waiting in a long queue, especially if you haven't got someone to save your place. The treats made everyone smile, and gave them some healing energy.

After signing lots of books, I needed some treats too. My right arm had dropped off. So I rummaged in my handbag with my left arm, to find a lipstick. With my left hand I applied thick, sticky, bubble-gum-pink lipstick to my lips. Without a compact mirror. I smiled. A mischievous clown smile. People held their books open at the first page, so I could kiss the page instead of signing it, like an adored and worshipped religious clown leader.

Woke up smiling and feeling holy. I thought my new idea for book signing was inspired, very innovative; though possibly more suitable for a glamour model who writes books, like Katie Price. I once saw her at one of her book signings, on her reality TV show, *What Katie Did Next*. After signing many books her hand nearly dropped off. She may like my book signing idea, her bee-sting-best-selling-lips would suit bright pink lipstick, because Katie loves to wear girlie pink. Maybe I'll contact her publisher. Maybe not.

Must promote my book. It would be much less effort, so much easier, if I could just dream about book signings. *Must* get a grip on reality. I would love a review in the winter edition of InterAction. Will ask Ben to email the Action for M.E. charity. It would be *so fantastic* to get a review in time for Christmas, but I think it may be too late for that. I will try. Nothing ventured, nothing strained.

It's too late to ask the M.E. Association for a review, their autumn edition of M.E. Essential is out next month. I'll ask Ben to email the man in charge of editing and advertising, Tony Britton, next year. A review or advertisement, mid October, would be *perfect* timing for a witchy book, just before Halloween.

Oh God. I may get awful reviews, it *is* a rather eccentric book. Will *anyone* want to read a book about a witch who has M.E.? Fans of J. K. Rowling's wonderful Harry Potter books, possibly. I will have to keep my fingers crossed. My broomsticks crossed too. Must remember to ask Ben to email Action for M.E. soon, I have a memory like a leaky cauldron.

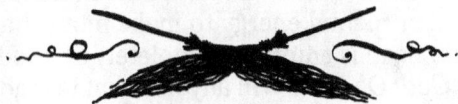

Will anyone want to spend £6.99 on a book? It *is* a lot of money when you have M.E., rely on benefit, and need your spare pennies for supplements. Supplements like Ginkgo Biloba and Echinacea; treatments like cranio sacral therapy; and books like Living With M.E., a self help guide by Dr. Charles Shepherd. *Also* reading is very tiring for most people with M.E.

I'm going to have nightmares, *I just know it*. I once knew a teacher who was so stressed, he often dreamt of a stick of white chalk chasing him. I will dream of stripy red and black Staedtler sharp-pointy-pencils, and gloomy green Berol italic pens, chasing me in freezing dark-inky-blue waters. I will find myself in the depths of Loch Ness. The monster will bite off my right arm, because I'm a silly author who writes about a witch feeding Nessie chocolate, so that he will sing to her.

I also write about Scottish dragons who like you to give them whisky, and tell them jokes about English, Irish and Scottish dragons going into a pub. Of course you can't tell those jokes to a Welsh dragon, because he will feel left out and probably fry your head off.

Saturday 4th

The proof copy of *Love & Best Witches* arrived from the printer this morning. Looks fine. Not too heavy for tired hands to pick up. Great. Nice, shiny cover. Magical-midnight-purpley-blue. Beautifully printed. Easy-on-the-eye creamy paper. Big type. Brilliant. My drawings look OK too. Very black. Verity black. Very bold. *Very* witchy. Wonderful.

Yes. I'm happy.

Well, I *think* I'm happy. I just wish I'd drawn that witch's hat a bit better and her cloak a little more billowy.... a waning moon would have looked better than a full moon in the midnight sky, although my constellations look OK.... there should be a comma there.... this drawing would have looked better a little bigger.... not sure that exclamation mark is necessary there.... that drawing should have been smaller.... possibly.... the cat's whiskers are too curly.... that didn't need a border really.... could have put more shading there.... the list of herb teas is too long.... that cat's tail is too short.... the candle smoke should have been drawn with dots.... but overall it's OK.... haven't got any more physical or mental energy to make more changes anyway.... my leaky cauldron head is empty.... completely drained.

Oh God! Oh God! Will anyone want to read it? Will anyone want to buy it? I will purchase lots of copies from Epic Press for friends and family. Maybe send copies to my witchy friends at Halloween, an ideal Halloween gift – it will soon be that time of year. I could send copies to friends and family for Christmas.

Good idea.

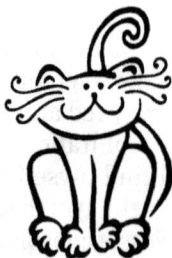

Sunday 5th

Today I feel floppy. Very floppy, worn out and useless, like the elastic in my old faded scrunchies. My sleepy-blue, weary-grey and bored-out-of-my-brain-brown scrunchies. I'm exhausted from all the mixed feelings of shiny-new-book-joy, I've-done-it-at-last-euphoria, and awful-author-anxiety.

Author anxiety brings to mind the pre-party nerves I experienced when I hosted a party in the eighties, many years before I became ill with M.E......

You send out the invitations, neatly written in your best I'm-a-confident-host writing, on jolly-party-invite paper from **WH Smith**. Make mix-tapes of rockin'-party-dancin' music, then spend hours in the kitchen preparing perfect-party-pastry foods and cheese cakes. Cheesecakes with a lovely crunchy base and arty-fruity-topping; mandarins and raspberries in a spiral pattern.

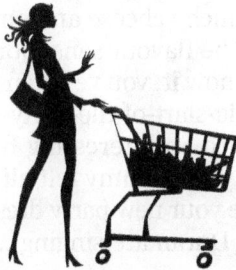

In Sainsbury's, you plod around purchasing party plates and paper napkins, cocktail sticks, drinks, mixers, delicious crispy crunchy delights and dips. On the day you make sandwiches with tasty fillings, cut into neat triangles. Then you stick cubes of cheddar, tiny onions, and pineapple chunks on cocktail sticks.

The day before, you whizzed around like a house-proud-maniac, making the house clean, tidy and welcoming, and telling yourself you feel fine. Not nervous. *Absolutely fine.* Fine, fine, fine.

When you've laid all the food out perfectly on party plates on the day, and poured crispy delights into party bowls; you pour yourself into your crispy new cotton marshmallow-pink party dress. You've never worn pink before. You feel quite girly and daring. Your hair is big and candy-floss fluffy, it took bloomin' ages to get it like that. Lots of gel. Lots of hair spray. Lots of blow-dry and back-combing. You have

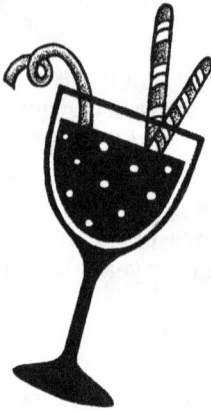

sparkling party eyes, flirty-flamingo-pink lips and nails to match. You pour yourself a well deserved glass of Merlot, to settle the first-half-hour-hostess-with-the-mostest-nerves.

During the first half hour the house is too quiet. Too empty. No party people yet. No music. You put on one of your mix-tapes, plump the cushions *again* and polish a cheese plant leaf you missed, with a party paper napkin. Then you polish off a cheese-and-silverskin-onion-on-a-stick, or two. Spandau Ballet are singing.... *Gold.... always believe in your soul....* You dance a little to get into the I'm-a-super-party-princess-mood. Then you notice your wine glass is empty.

In the kitchen you pour yourself a *small* glass of wine, you don't want to be crawling to the front door to greet your guests. Trying not to panic that no-one will turn up, that *everyone will have forgotten,* you nibble a crisp. A beautiful big crunchy cheese and onion crisp. Your favourite. It melts on your tongue. The flavour sensation making you feel better.

Before you know it, you've eaten a whole bowl of crisps, to crunch away the unbearable-start-of-the-party-seconds. You should have had your baked potato with an interesting filling for dinner, but you were feeling anxious and your tummy felt all tight. Although this was quite a good thing, because your new party dress was tight and you could only just fit into it. Duran Duran are singing..... *juices like wine..... and I'm hungry like the wolf.....*

The kitchen clock seems to be ticking a lot louder than usual. TICK..... TOCK..... TICK..... DON'T..... PAN..... ICK..... You find another packet of crisps and pour them into the empty party bowl. The crisps you've eaten have made you thirsty, so..... maybe..... just one more small drink before the guests arrive. Ooops! The glass is full to the brim.

You find yourself on your hands and knees by the front door. Not because you have drunk too much wine. *No, nooo.* Not because you are waiting to worship your first guest, although you feel a little that way inclined. It's just that one of the cats has been sick. A delightful fur-ball, perfectly placed on the welcome mat, where your first guest will tread in it.

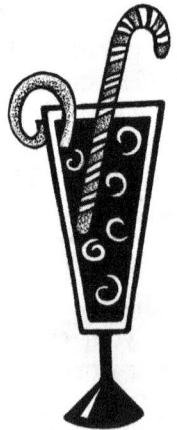

6

When you've cleaned up the mess with kitchen roll, you notice a hole in your tights. On the right knee. Must have been where you knelt on the spiky rush mat. This look will not match your pretty party dress. It's pink, not punk. The phone rings.

The answering machine takes the message. Your best friend Rosie is *really really* sorry that she can't make it to your party because her baby-sitter, for the twins, Thomas and Jerry, has let her down. You wonder if Thomas has chased Jerry out of the house, and Rosie is running around the garden after them; must be the wine making your imagination run wild. You are *very very* disappointed, because you were so sure she would be the first to arrive. Even if it were just you and her, you'd have a great-giggly-girly time.

Forty-five minutes have passed. You crunch more cheese and onion crisps, and nibble a couple more cheese-and-onion-on-a-stick delicacies. Then you pour yourself another *small* glass of wine. Maybe you should turn the music up, so that you can't hear the kitchen clock ticking away the pre-party-minutes. You are sure it's ticking louder on purpose..... TICK..... TOCK..... TICK..... CAT'S..... BEEN..... SICK..... MORE..... CRISPS..... QUICK.

In your bedroom you hunt for a pair of clean ladder-free tights. The Bangles are singing..... *Just another manic Monday..... wish it was Sunday..... that's my fun day..... my I don't have to run day.....* You find a new pair of tights, still in the packet. Not opened yet. Hurrah! Then realise you need to go to the loo.

In the bathroom you notice a crimson wine stain down the front of your new crispy clean party-pink dress. How did that happen? You blame Duran Duran for making you feel *all dancy*. Your gorgeous candy-floss hair is going flat and your face is flushed. You look like you're halfway through the evening already.

Feeling hot, in a huff, and hurt that your best friend can't make it to the party, you take off all your clothes and search for something to wear that doesn't need ironing. Your best jeans will do. Maybe that new white tee-shirt. Maybe the little black dress, to suit your black mood.

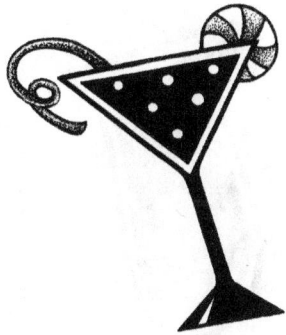

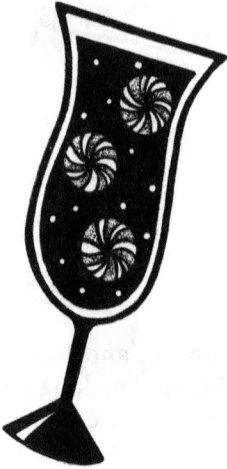

Suddenly you feel very tired. You just want to curl up in bed and go to sleep. Wham are singing..... *Wake me up before you go go*..... In the bathroom you feel you need more than just a *wee,* so you open the bathroom window, your guests don't want to be greeted by a smelly bathroom. A cool summer breeze makes you sneeze, and your party make-up starts to run, lipstick smudges and you look like you've been crying. You shut the window. You feel like crying. You sit on the toilet singing..... *it's my party and I'll cry if I want to..... cry if I want to..... cry if I want to.....* You went to so much trouble to make the bathroom clean and freshly scented with pot-pourri, and put out pretty pink guest towels.

The pink towels and rose scented pot-pourri would have matched your party dress and perfume. The sort of thing your mother would notice; not your cool party pals wearing shoulder pads and Lycra, cerise leopard print and big shiny accessories, to match their big hair.

As you sit naked and shivering on the toilet, you feel that you *know, just know;* your first guest will arrive *and* you won't hear the doorbell because you forgot to turn the music down. ABC are singing..... *shoot that poison arrow to my heart, shoot that poison arrow*..... you want someone to shoot you with a poison arrow.

As you pull on your jeans, you think you hear the doorbell. You have a feeling it's Gail and Gareth, who have travelled a long distance and will probably need the bathroom *right away.*

* * * * * *

I imagine, when you have a book published, you experience the first three-quarters of an hour pre-party nerves for six months. If you are lucky, at the end of the six months, you receive a lovely letter from your publisher on posh paper, and a lovelier cheque, making you feel like royalty.

Ben emailed Epic Press tonight to give them the go-ahead with the book. The book I have actually completed. It's done. Oh God. *This is it.* No going back.

September

Monday 6th

6.30 p.m.   Ben arrives home with the weekly shopping from Tesco.

6.33 p.m.   Under the bananas, bread and soya milk, I spy with my tired little eye, two treats. A bar of Galaxy Bubbles and a of box Maltesers. *Lovely*. Just what I need. Chocolate. Fortunately Ben loves chocolate too, so I'm not tempted to devour the whole lot myself in one evening. Something that would take no effort at all. Somehow chocolate just seems to fly magically through the air towards my mouth.

6.34 p.m.   Deliciously divine..... Silky smooth..... Aromatic and addictive..... Tempting and tantalising.

If I were a headmaster, I would get rid of the history teacher and get a chocolate teacher instead and my pupils would study a subject that affected all of them

ROALD DAHL

It's not that chocolates are a substitute for love..... love is a substitute for chocolate

MIRANDA INGRAM

Chocolate is the best cure for author anxiety

VERITY RED

6.35 p.m.   Author anxiety has lifted.

6.36 p.m.   The bubbles in Maltesers and an Aero bar, give the witch in my book an extra lift when she flies to Tesco on her broomstick. She needs the extra lift if the carrier bag hanging on her broomstick is heavy with tins of cat food. She would *love* Galaxy Bubbles. I couldn't mention them in my book because they have only just appeared on the market, I saw them advertised in Weekly Wife last week.

6.38 p.m.   Ben has bought kitchen roll with a new magical star design. Lemon yellow and plum purple stars. The witch in my book would love that too.

6.39 p.m.   I want to add the Galaxy Bubbles and magical kitchen roll to my story, but it's too late now. The book is done. *Completely completed.* Need more chocolate.

6.40 p.m.   Mmm..... Celestial..... Sublime..... Sinful.....

6.50 p.m.   I'm not hungry for my dinner now.

6.55 p.m.   Ben munches Quorn burgers, chips and peas.

7.00 p.m.   Find my old mix-tapes of eighties music on cassette.

If music be the food of love, I'll have a concerto and chips please

VERITY RED

7.05 p.m.   Burgers, chips, peas
Concerto, chips, please

Think I feel a verse coming on. Will need more chocolate to activate creative brain cells.

7.10 p.m.   I recline (like an Egyptian queen) with my tabby cat, Cleopatra, and nibble the last of the Galaxy..... luscious..... decadent..... irresistible. Right Said Fred sing..... *I'm too sexy for my cat.....*

7.35 p.m.   Ben gives me another surprise. Two hair scrunchies he bought in Tesco. Wonderful *tight* elastic. Navy blue and bottle green back-to-school scrunchies.

7.36 p.m.   Oh joy! I can tie my long hair back, very tightly. My needed-a-wash-days-ago-but-I-haven't-had-the-energy hair.

7.37 p.m.   I will wear the navy blue scrunchie first, because that was the colour of my school uniform. What fun. When you have M.E. the little things mean a lot. The only problem is I'm suffering with that back-to-school feeling. And I've just handed in my 153 page creative writing project, *Love & Best Witches*. Will I get a B plus or a C minus? Or a big F for failure? Oh God.

Tuesday 7th

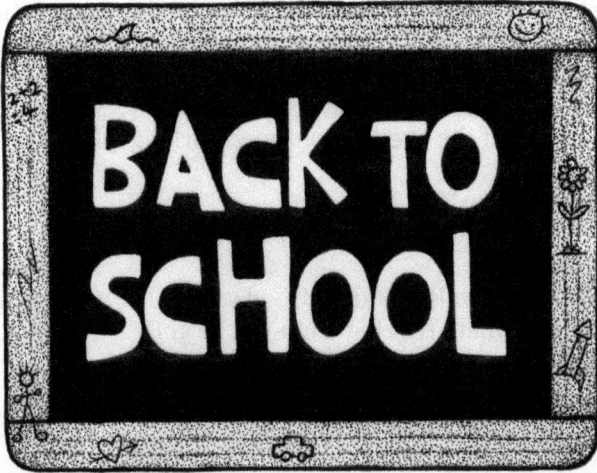

My back-to-school feelings continued today when a leaflet from Sainsbury's arrived with the post, advertising their half price products. There was a picture of a child's chalk board with back-to-school written on it. Identity Direct catalogue arrived too: back-to-school personalised pens and pencils, sports bags, back packs, lunch boxes, clothing labels.....

I liked the little pictures you can have printed on the clothing name labels, in bright rainbow colours. There's a lovely choice: elephants, dinosaurs, bees, flowers, butterflies, smiley faces, cars, skull and cross bones, fairies.....

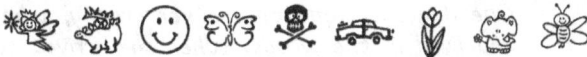

It would be good if there were clothing name labels for grown-ups too. Maybe a picture of a teapot, wine glass, cat, dog, smiley sunshine..... this could be useful if you have M.E. and you have one of those days when you can barely remember your name or what day it is.

The witch in my book would have liked name labels with pictures of bats, pumpkins, cauldrons, black cats, moons, stars or pentacles. It's too late to put new bits in my book. I must stop my brain wanting to continue to work on it, checking for errors and spelling mistakes..... maybe removing that paragraph..... re-drawing the witch on her broomstick..... re-drawing the cat on her broomstick.....

10.00 a.m.   In bathroom washing face.
              I think I'll write a short children's story to take my mind off the *need* to continue working on my book.

10.02 a.m.   Brushing teeth.
              Thinking of children's stories.

10.03 a.m.   Little Red Riding Hood said to her granny..... 'Oh, Granny, what great big teeth you've got!'

10.04 a.m.   Need to tinkle.
              Sit on loo.
              Need a title.

10.06 a.m.   Think of title: Verity Red Riding Hood.
              There will be no wolf with big teeth, just a dear old granny with a big heart.

10.26 a.m.   In bath.

              Once upon a time there was a little girl. Her name was Verity Red Riding Hood. Verity was always tired because she had M.E.

10.28 a.m.   Wash with lavender soap.

              One day she went to see her granny, who was a witch and lived in the woods. When she arrived at the cottage

12

she was so tired that granny tucked her up in a lovely warm bed. The bed had a big patchwork quilt; beautiful soft greens and lilacs, and smelling of lavender.

1.00 p.m.   In kitchen.
Making tasty cheese and tomato sandwich for lunch.

Granny always had something tasty bubbling in her cauldron. That day she had made a special soup that would make Verity Red Riding Hood feel better. It smelt very delicious. Carrot, orange and coriander soup.

1.10 p.m.   Staring out of kitchen window.

When Verity had finished her soup, she fell into a deep sleep for a week. She dreamt of dancing in the woods with the pixies and fairies. Singing, laughing, and playing leap-frog with the frogs.

3.15 p.m.   I wake up after catnap with my cats.

When Verity awoke she felt much better and full of energy. She was so overjoyed, she gave her granny a big hug and kiss on her rosy cheek. Then she ran all the way home and lived happily ever after.

THE END

3.20 p.m.   I mentioned carrot, orange and coriander soup in my witchy book. I wish I'd put the recipe in too.

3.30 p.m.   Find recipe in my witchy cook book.

1 lb thinly sliced carrots
1 thinly sliced onion
½ oz butter
1 pint water
1 tsp crushed coriander seeds
Juice of 4 large oranges (or ½ pint of orange juice)
Thinly sliced rind of 1 orange

Fry the carrots and onions gently in butter for around ten minutes. Add water and coriander seeds, bring to the boil and simmer gently for fifteen minutes. Blend really thoroughly. Add the orange juice and rind. Cook gently for a further five minutes and taste to see whether it needs salt. Cool thoroughly and chill for at least an hour before serving.

3.31 p.m.   The witchy cook says this is a great energy-giver, whether on a physical or a magical plane. I haven't made a witchy soup for years. *Must do.* When I have some spare energy, whether on a physical or a magical plane.

4.23 p.m.   Read about getting the kids back to school in Weekly Wife. Wendy's best buys were the enchanted pink pencil case, blue shark pencil case, and hands-off-my-lunch lunch box. Wendy also told me to look effortlessly chic, yet feel oh-so comfy in drapey jersey fabrics; shades of pistachio, beige and sand. I'd rather look effortlessly droopy in my old cardies, thanks Wendy. In shades of limp lettuce, pale parchment, and tired-out-taupe.

Wednesday 8th

I awoke to a beautiful bright sunny morning. The yolk in my boiled egg, late summer sunshine yellow; my slice of toast, crunchy and brown as autumn leaves.

Late morning, I plodded outside into the garden with my tupperware box of peanuts, a slice of old thick crusty wholemeal bread resting on top. After I had filled the bird table I held my pale, tired face up to the sun and warmed my mind with soothing sunbeams. The back-to-school-navy-blues lifted and drifted high, up into the sky. The serene September-blue sky.

As I slowly wandered back indoors, a cool gentle breeze whispered in my ear of falling leaves, and did I know I had dried egg yolk on my cheek.

Late afternoon I read my stars in Weekly Wife. Cosmic Colin said I had lots to catch up on this week, and to make sure I paced myself. Also I should do something fun on the 8th.

Colin is *so* clever. How does he know I have M.E. and pacing is one of the most important ways to cope with the illness?

What shall I do for fun? *I know!* Ben bought an egg slicer at the weekend. If I run a teaspoon over the little wires it sounds like a miniature harp. A harp for fairies. I will practice playing the egg slicer tonight.

That will be fun.

Thursday 9th

My copy of InterAction from A.F.M.E. arrived today. Once I started to read it I couldn't put it down. I shed a tear when I read about children who have M.E. Quite a few tears really. They dripped all over the page making it soggy.

An amusing article by Diane Shortland made me cackle like an old witch. She wrote about what it's like when you emerge into the outside world after years of being housebound with M.E. and so much has changed. I could *so* identify with her observations, and recalled the time I wandered into Mothercare in search of a little cute baby-grow. I found myself in a record shop full of young lads, wearing cool teenage-grow jeans and I'm-a-serious-rock-star tee-shirts.

The A.F.M.E. Christmas cards looked nice. Decided to order the bargain pack and Christmas paper.

1.30 p.m.   Sent two text messages. One to Ben, the other to my friend Jayne who has M.E.

B - CAN U GET DE-CAF TEA ON YOUR WAY HOME - THANX X

HI JAYNE, HOPE U COPED OK WITH YOR BIG MOVE ON WED - WISHIN U LOTS OF ENERGY 2 RECOVER - HUGS XUX

Jayne has moved out of her parents house, to live with her boyfriend in South London. Her family have never understood or *believed* how ill she is. At times they have been very cruel to her. My heart has been breaking for her, for years. There are no words to describe how *utterly relieved, tearfully relieved,* I feel that she has escaped.

No words.

9.00 p.m.   *Coronation Street* was good tonight. Ken Barlow's son Lawrence turned up on his doorstep. The son is William Roache's (who plays Ken) *real life* son, Linus. Lawrence tells Ken he has a grandson, James. James is William Roache's *other* real life son, whose *real* name is James. There is a family dispute because James is estranged from Lawrence. I so enjoyed the family resemblance and I'm looking forward to seeing the grandson, the other *real life* son.

An exciting evening.

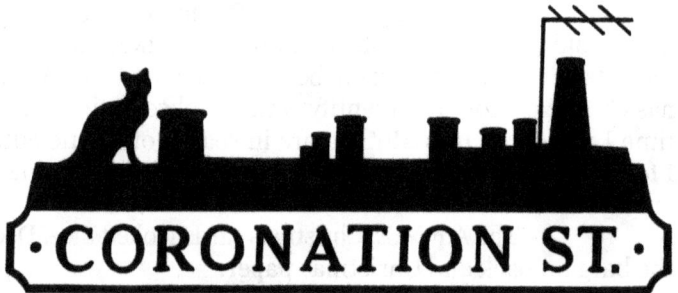

Friday 10th

11.25 a.m.   Two parcels (Christmas gifts) have arrived.
              Goody! Love getting parcels.

11.26 a.m.   Study shapes of parcels to prolong the love-getting-parcels-euphoria. One of the parcels is long and thin, that must be the 'Wizards and dragons' calendars I ordered from ACE catalogue. The other parcel is soft and squishy, must be the knitted slippers I ordered from The Original Gift Company.

11.29 a.m.   The pictures on the calendars are sparkly and magical. Lots of scary, red and green dragons with enormous wings, talons, and big pointy teeth. Lots of eccentric looking long bearded wizards with flowing robes and huge pointy hats.

11.32 a.m. Feeling poetic.....

Pointy hats
Flowing robes
Unicorns and cats
And toads
Teeth and talons
Nostrils aflare
Bats caught up in
Wizards hair

11.34 a.m. The witch in my book loves wizards and dragons. She would like this calendar. I keep forgetting my book is done. My memory is like the leakiest cauldron with a big crack in the side, and all the witchy broth is seeping out. Have to keep reminding myself the book is done. *Done, finished, completed.*

11.35 a.m. The calendars are for my Harry Potter loving friends.

11.36 a.m. The knitted slippers are for my friends who have M.E. Like me, they live in their slippers. Good colours. Gentle grey, soft blue, pale pink and lilac. Restful shades for sleepy eyes and minds.

11.50 a.m. Sip herbal-green peppermint tea. Stare sleepily out of the kitchen window, admiring the soft greys and pinks on the feathers of the wood pigeons.

12.46 p.m. Text from Jayne:

HI, WE FINALLY MOVED LAST NITE – MY DAD HAS DISOWNED ME FOR NOW, BUT I DON-T CARE, I-M FREE – HAPPY – HOW-RE YOU? WE-RE STILL GETTING THINGS SORTED OUT – I-M SO EXHAUSTED, BUT HAPPY – THANK U FOR ALL UR SUPPORT – HUGS XXX

12.47 p.m.   I replied:

OOH, HURRAH – YOU-VE FINALLY ESCAPED, I-M OVER
THE MOON – THANX FOR LETTIN ME KNOW SO SOON –
KNOW HOW U MUST BE FEELIN – HEALING HUGS XXVXX

7.00 p.m.   Watching the romantic comedy, *Runaway Bride*. Julia
Roberts is such a pretty woman.

7.35 p.m.   Feeling very tired and pale. I would make a good drift-
away-ghostly-bride. On a bad day – a perfect corpse bride.

Saturday 11th

8.30 a.m.   Wake up to noisy builders next door, hammering to the
beat of heavy rock music.

8.45 a.m.   Sounds like they are throwing heavy rocks into the skip
outside now. Peer out of the window. They are removing
fireplaces.

9.05 a.m.   My new neighbour, the other side of our terraced house,
is banging doors to head-banging-music. Sounds like his
young girlfriend has left him again.

10.00 a.m.   My neighbours, both sides, have moved recently. Many
people in our street have moved recently. Is there something
I should know? I'm having visions of an earthquake, and
our whole street falling into a big dark hole in the ground.
Is it time we moved?

10.01 a.m.   Just the thought of all the upheaval, all the packing, makes
me feel ill, very exhausted.

10.02 a.m.   I don't like the word move. Or movement. Stillness.....
staying still..... silence..... solitude..... serenity..... soft.....
soothing..... spiritual.....
Words I love.

10.35 a.m.   Have returned to bed, after feeding and watering my cats, the wildlife, and myself.

10.36 a.m.   My little grey cat, Mary, is cuddled up to me. So soft..... sweet..... soothing..... silky fur. We are serene and silent. No movement, just the twitching of whiskers and paws. Peaceful, loving solitude. Her tiny chest rising and falling, as she dreams beautiful cat dreams.

10.37 a.m.   Purrdita, my tabby, is perched on my shoulder. As always, purring. She yawns a huge tabby yawn. I yawn, a huge human yawn.

10.38 a.m.   Purring is the most comforting sound in the world.

10.39 a.m.   Apart from the sound of unwrapping a bar of Galaxy Bubbles.

10.40 a.m.   Cleopatra, the stray tabby I've recently taken in, snores at my feet. A soft contented tabby snore.

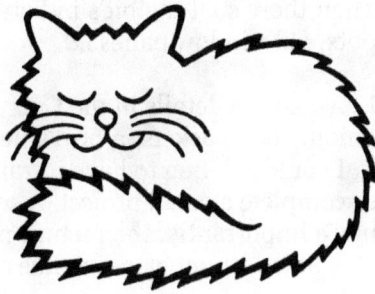

6.00 p.m.   Leafing through TV mag.
There's a programme on at 8.00 p.m. — Britain's Secret Fat Cats. Strange. A programme about people who keep their overweight moggies a secret.

6.01 p.m.   Oh. It's not about cats.

Financial journalist Ben Lawrence looks into whether the major beneficiaries of the government's spending cuts are private out sourcing companies.

That sounds like a bundle of laughs.

6.02 p.m.   I know!
I've got a jigsaw puzzle to complete. A 500 piece picture of Crazy Cats. I think they're in a garden. Or a shed (the cats, not the puzzle).

6.17 p.m.   Have found puzzle!
Crazy Cats..... in the Potting Shed. I've already completed most of the cats in the window. Cat sleeping in an old deckchair. Cat on a box. Cat in a box. Cats sitting in a thread-bare chair. Cat curled up with flower pots.

6.18 p.m.   I just need to piece together the black cat in the window with white paws, tabby cat peering through cat flap and white cat sitting by rusty watering can.

6.19 p.m.   Then there's all the bit's in between; floorboards, flower pots, old window panes.....

6.20 p.m.   I love all the details in the Crazy Cats picture. A dried up onion, seed packets, a bird's nest..... When I've finished it, I could ask Ben to have it framed for me. It will be *fun* to complete a small project. A sense of *achievement*. But, more importantly, the picture makes me smile. I cannot look at it without grinning like a crazy cat.

6.21 p.m.   I will learn to love jigsaw puzzles. I *really will try*. Like the time when I learned to love swede, because it was the only organic vegetable Ben could find in Sainsbury's.

Sunday 12th

Last night I put together an enormous chocolate Crazy Cats jigsaw puzzle in a field. Every piece was as large as the average square sofa cushion, thick as a big slab of Galaxy chocolate, and wrapped in foil; with a part-of-the-puzzle picture printed on the front. I could not eat any of the fifty piece puzzle until I had completed it.

When I had finally finished my task, I lay on the grass exhausted. I stared at the stars twinkling in the midnight sky, imagining galaxies far, far away. Then a dragon appeared flying overhead. He breathed fire and the puzzle melted away.

I woke up feeling hot, bothered, and with a crazy-cat-craving for creamy Galaxy chocolate. I wanted a chocolate egg in an egg cup and chocolate spread on toast for breakfast. I wondered why I had dreamt of a jigsaw made of chocolate. My mind was puzzled for a moment, then I pieced together the memories of the last two days. I recalled seeing a Santa Claus chocolate jigsaw in a Christmas gift catalogue on Friday. On Saturday, I had flicked through *Love & Best Witches* with a critical eye, and wished I had drawn one of the dragons breathing more fire.

12.10 p.m.   Before Ben flew out the front door to do some shopping, he called up the stairs, 'Text me if you can think of anything you want from Sainsbury's.'

12.11 p.m.   YES, GALAXY BUBBLES – THANX X

1.05 p.m.   *Delicious!*
              The dreamy Galaxy bubbles have enlivened me. I've started piecing together more of the Crazy Cats in the potting shed puzzle.

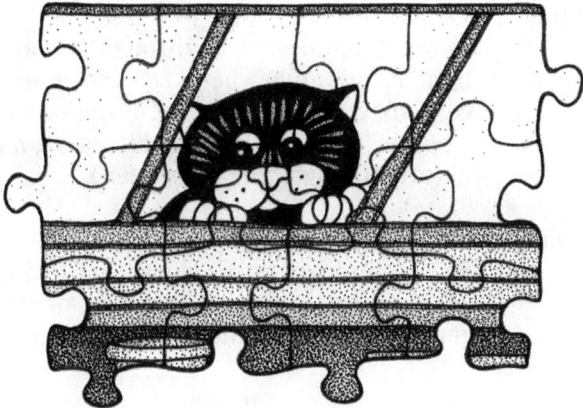

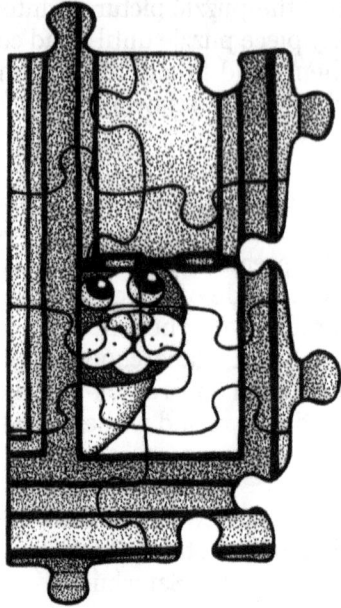

1.55 p.m.   *Great!*
I've found old boots, a rake, flower pots, ball of string, black cat with white paws in window, tabby cat peering through cat flap, and white cat sitting by rusty watering can.

2.02 p.m.   *Cackle!*
I love the cat peering in through the cat flap. It never fails to make me smile when I see one of my cats sitting at the cat flap, either looking out at the rain (wishing it would stop) or looking in, and making a big *meeooww* to be let in (even though the flap is open).

2.35 p.m.   *Hurrah!*
Have found gardening gloves, gardening fork and spade, dried onion, bird house, wilting plant in chamber pot, geranium in pot, spider web in window, and bird's nest.

2.36 p.m.   *Ouch!*
My neck is starting to seize up. So are my shoulders and back. My eyes are as sleepy as a contented, well fed, cat in a potting shed.

2.37 p.m.   *Sigh!*
I just have to find a few pieces of dusty old floorboard and half a rusty tin bucket.

2.41 p.m.   *Well done me!*
I've completed another project. Will award myself more Galaxy chocolate. I'm grinning like a crazy cat, with chocolate on her paws and a stiff collar round her neck.

4.20 p.m.   Cleopatra is purring on my lap. It's a faint purr, but it's gradually getting louder as the days go by. She's very thin and scabby, but I'll soon have her nicely rounded and contented, with a shiny coat. Her white paws look a little yellow, like they are nicotine stained. Have those alley cats been encouraging her into bad habits?

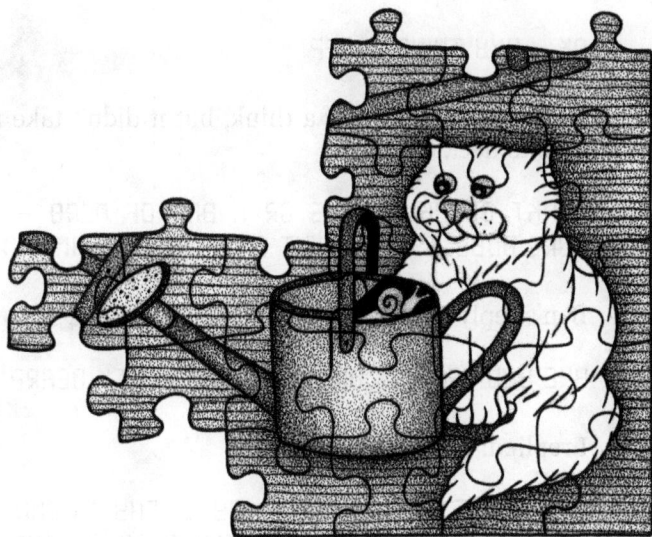

4.22 p.m.   I gently stroke her long tail. Because she's a girl she enjoys a bit of rub-tail-therapy. I stroke her paws. They will soon be healthy-cat-paw white. White as the cat paws in my jigsaw puzzle.

4.30 p.m.   My claws need trimming. I'm sure since I got M.E. they have been growing faster. My toe claws too. Maybe it's the copious amounts of oil of evening primrose oil I consume every week.

4.33 p.m.   The soft rumbly sound of purring, pitter-patter of rain-drops on the window pane, and the whistling wind, is *so relaxing*. Cleopatra's wind is not so relaxing, but it makes me smile. How can such a small sweet cat, with a tiny bum, make such a big stinky-bomb-smell. *Phew!*

4.36 p.m.   Text Ben, he popped back into town about half an hour ago:

              JUST REMEMBERED, WE NEED MORE CAT LITTER

4.39 p.m.   Ben replied:

              OK - ANY THING ELSE?

4.40 p.m.   I replied after a bit of a think, but it didn't take me too long to decide:

              A PKT OF MALTESERS OR A BAR OF AERO - I NEED MORE BUBBLES FOR A BIT OF A LIFT - THANX   X

4.41 p.m.   Ben's reply made me smile:

              ARE YOU OFF OUT ON YOUR BROOMSTICK DEAR?

4.42 p.m.   I replied:

              OF COURSE - I'M MEETING MY WITCHY FRIEND JAYNE LATER, FOR A PINT OF BUTTER BEER AT THE LEAKY CAULDRON

4.45 p.m.	Cleopatra has the largest, most beautiful, sad, pale green and turquoise eyes I've ever seen. They look like they are outlined with khol, Egyptian-queen-style, and full of wondrous ancient Egyptian wisdom.
4.47 p.m.	I have a thousand piece jigsaw, somewhere, of Egyptian Pharaohs. This could be my new project. A new adventure in ancient Egypt. *How Lovely*. Piecing together all those little hieroglyphs will be such fun.
4.50 p.m.	I need to move now, sitting on this hard kitchen chair has made my bum go numb, and stiff as an Egyptian mummy. My tired face is still and solemn as Tutankhamun's mask.
4.51 p.m.	Mary is sitting on the kitchen worktop like a tiny grey sphinx. The sun has come out and my sun-catcher sparkles. Magical rainbow shades adorn Mary's fur. There must be a rainbow somewhere in the sky.
4.54 p.m.	I'm in the bedroom, staring out of the window, and admiring a perfect arch of radiant colours over our little town. A bow on mother nature's gift to us. The gift of life.
4.55 p.m.	I mention rainbows in my witchy book. I say very little, wish I'd said more. But the book is *done* now. *Completely completed* and printed.
4.56 p.m.	Gazing at the beauty of the rainbow, I feel poetic.

> *You can't have a rainbow*
> *Without the rain*
> *You can't have the love*
> *Without the pain*

Maybe the next verse will be something about a train..... or a plane..... or a stain..... inspiration is fading away softly, almost imperceptibly, like a rainbow.

I wish rainbows
Would stay longer in the sky
I wish I were a bird
With wings, and I could fly

Inspiration can be like a rainbow, it appears magically out of the blue, and fills you with wonderful bright colourful thoughts. When it fades you don't feel sad because it's still there, a delightful memory in the soft sky blue of your mind's eye.

5.25 p.m.   I'm wallowing in a warm bubble bath. Hubble Bubble Bath is the title of Chapter Eight in my book, in which the witch enjoys a hubble bubble bath. I wish I'd mentioned..... no I don't, *no, no, no,* the book is done, *completely completed.*

5.26 p.m.   I love to be surrounded by bubbles. Fluffy candy floss clouds, made up of millions of magical iridescent globes. Swirling rainbow spheres all around me, and the comforting sound of pop, pop, perfumed popping..... tiny scented explosions of wild berries and flowers.

5.27 p.m.   A bath-bomb sits on the side of my bath. It's from Lush, and called Dorothy; sky blue, with a pink, orange and yellow rainbow. The fragrance is so delightful; it makes my nose feel full of rainbows that drift up into my eyes, making them sparkle like pink champagne at a summer wedding..... a cluster of diamonds in springtime sunshine..... tears of joy, when in autumn you finally complete a jigsaw puzzle.

5.28 p.m.   I'm singing *Somewhere Over the Rainbow*, in my best Dorothy-off-to-see-the-wizard-of-Oz voice. I don't want to put the Dorothy bath bomb in my bath water. It will explode, fizzle away, dissolve and disappear completely into the bathtime blue, like a rainbow dissolving into a rainy day sky. I just like to pick it up, and enjoy the perfumed sensation making my nose sparkle.

5.30 p.m.   Sniff..... sniff.....sni*ffffffffff*

Rainbows have fallen
From the sky
Into the bubbles
Where I lie

5.32 p.m.   I love Judy Garland playing Dorothy in *The Wizard of Oz*. But I was a little disappointed to read recently, that her real name was Frances Ethel Gumm – like the time I found out Elton John's real name is Reg Dwight; and he told me, in his song, *Candle in the Wind*, that Marilyn Monroe's real name was Norma Jean.

5.33 p.m.   Recall a poem I wrote over ten years ago, in a bubble bath, when I first became ill with M.E.

Yesterday
All my bubbles
Seemed so far away
Now it looks as though
They're here to stay
Oh, I believe
In deodorant spray
Suddenly
I'm remembering
How it used to be
When I had
Oh, so much energy
Oh, I wish it
Was yesterday

Why I had to get ill
I don't know
The doctors couldn't say
I did something wrong
Now I long for
Yesterday

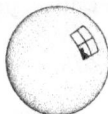

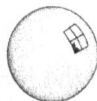

Yesterday
Life was such
An easy game to play
Now I need my bed
To hide away
Oh, I wish it
Was
Yesterday

I hoped dear John Lennon in pop star heaven and Sir Paul, wouldn't mind my new version of their song.

8.30 p.m.   Watching the film première of *Fool's Gold*. My hands are feeling too weak to pick up my mug of de-caf tea, but I feel inspired to pick up a pen.

Don't go chasing
Rainbows
In the pouring
Rain
You may find
The pot of gold
Will only
Cause you pain

When it's too heavy for you to pick up

Monday 13th

Two Christmas gift catalogues arrived from the R.S.P.C.A. and the N.S.P.C.C. The witch in my book supports the R.S.P.C.W. (The Royal Society for the Prevention of Cruelty to Witches). I've *actually* thought of my book *without* wanting to change something or put a new idea in. Progress at last.

12.15 p.m.   Love getting Christmas catalogues. It's such a pleasure to let my fingers do the walking, and I don't have to queue with tired feet, my toes all scrunched up in winter boots. No crossing roads, freezing at the service till or bus stops. I can flutter through the pages like a joyful butterfly, alighting on anything colourful that catches my eye.

12.25 p.m. I think I'll order the delightful silk scarf for auntie, adorned with many colourful butterflies. The catalogue says it rests effortlessly across your shoulders.
Rest..... Effortlessly..... wonderful words.

12.30 p.m. Very tempted to order the tin of chocolate heaven, and large box of chocolate perfection for myself. I will not be tempted. But do I need some note cards. Twenty assorted, with pictures of wildlife, will be perfect. It's *so much* easier to write to pen friends on a note card, especially if the picture is inspiring; a beautiful fox, badger or blue tit. Faced with a blank sheet of paper, my tired mind just goes completely blank. I don't know what to write, where to start, how to string a few words together to make a sentence. Where do you start? When your life is so full of exciting adventures; like, the day before yesterday you actually climbed the mountain of stairs in one go. The day before that, you actually managed to dry yourself after your bath. Well, maybe not your whole body. But you didn't have to lie on the floor for an hour, to find some energy to dry yourself.

12.34 p.m. HOT! HOT! HOT! Chilli jam, seriously hot vulcan mustard, Caribbean hot sauce, and sweet chilli in a big red box, looks an ideal gift for Ben.

12.35 p.m. THE BLACK BOX; Catherine wheels, menthol liquorice pellets, liquorice and aniseed drops, Pontefract cakes, liquorice sticks, Australian liquorice and magic wands. Wonderful for my liquorice loving friend.
The witch in my book has liquorice wands at her parties, so I'm not wishing I'd put that in the book, hurrah!

12.36 p.m. FOUR CHRISTMAS PUDDINGS; Infused with Guinness and suitable for vegetarians, will make a suitably delicious gift for my Guinness loving vegetarian friend.

12.40 p.m.   FLUFFY BED SOCKS; Embroidered with cuddly bears. Pale lavender, fluffy-snowflake-white and soft-strawberry-ice-cream-pink. A perfect gift for friends who are bedridden with M.E.

12.43 p.m.   PESTLE AND MORTAR; A useful gift, for a witchy friend to grind her herbs. The witch in my book doesn't have one. Do I care? No, *the book is done.*

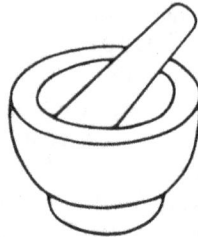

1.00 p.m.   Fill in order form for Christmas cards and Christmas paper from A.F.M.E.

3.00 p.m.   Fill mug with hot water, and enjoy the aroma of peppermint tea.

3.03 p.m.   Sitting outside in the warm sunshine, watching the breeze making the trees sway like boats in a harbour. A pale brown sycamore seed, the shape of a moth's wing, flutters down helicopter-style into my tea, and floats like a wooden rowing boat in dark seaweed-green waters.

3.04 p.m.   My broomstick is leaning against the fence, soon it will be covered with fallen leaves; they will keep it warm for the winter (so I won't have too much trouble getting it started for a flight in the springtime).

7.45 p.m.   Ben emails A.F.M.E. to ask if they will review my book in InterAction, in time for Christmas. Fingers crossed.

7.46 p.m.   Broomsticks crossed.

Tuesday 14th

Tuesday is gig night for Ben. He performs with his mate Paul at the Mexxa Mexxa restaurant in town. They play guitar and call themselves the Avocado Pair.

The apple-green hand towels I recently ordered from La Redoute catalogue look avocado-ish, and match our avocado-green bathroom suite. I commented to Ben that he is a very lucky boy, his towels and bathroom suite match the name of his duo. He gave me one of his *looks*.

I have ordered apple and bracken-green stripy bath towels from La Redoute. They will match the leaves on the spider plants in our bathroom *and* Ben's toothbrush. He will be simply enthralled. He doesn't know I will soon be ordering a bracken-green, high tufted bath mat. Very soft and absorbent. Super-soft quality. Washable at sixty degrees and a hundred percent cotton. I will keep this a secret for now, the excitement will be too much for him.

Before Ben went out to his gig at the restaurant, he checked his emails. Clare, the deputy editor of InterAction, had replied to his request about reviewing my book. She said the book sounded lovely and she would really like to see a copy. Clare also said she had a stack of books to consider, but will get back to him a.s.a.p.

ME: *Oooh! Wonderful!* And how kind of Clare to reply so soon, I can imagine how busy she must be.

BEN: *Yeah!......................................Right I'm off.*

ME: Have a good gig Mr Avocado.

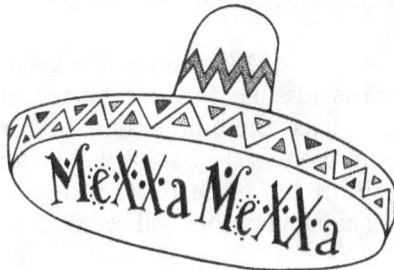

Wednesday 15th

11.45 a.m.   I'm not so happy today. *Not happy at all.* I'm *very angry.* Horrified. *Inert.* An indignant individual. Do I feel a verse coming on with lots of alliteration? *NO.* I'm illiterate and inert with indignation and indigestion.

11.48 a.m.   I felt really happy last night; why, *why, why,* does this letter have to arrive today and spoil it all. WHY.

11.49 a.m.   Our borough council has written, to say their waste collection team plans to install a recycling site in the small car park next to our street. The five recycling skips for clothes and bottles will be located opposite our house, a stones-throw-away. Or maybe I should say, a bottles-throw-away. Oh Great. That is just *wonderful.* It will be like a rubbish tip in our front garden, because we don't have a front garden, just a small road, then the car park.

11.51 a.m.   Just *brilliant.*
              Crashing and smashing sounds at all hours. Then there's the noise of the collection lorries, their entrance *right opposite* our house. There's a lot of old people in our street that need their peace in the day. Like me. I'm not old but I'm getting there fast; I feel like I've aged ten years in the past few hours, and my face is full of anger wrinkles.

11.52 a.m.   After a hard day's work, the other residents in our street will need their peace in the evenings. Like Ben.

12.34 p.m.   When you have M.E. you need to keep calm and peaceful as much as possible. How will I ever feel calm and peaceful again. At least the builders next door will be gone one day soon, the recycling skips will be forever. I'm sipping peppermint tea to ease my indignant indigestion, and thinking about pets; they will be frightened by the noise.

12.35 p.m.   Sip....... Sip....... *Slurp.*

32

Daydreaming about living by the sea; the sound of seagulls and waves crashing on the shore. Silently sailing ships in the distance.

12.36 p.m. Trying not to think of the sound of bottles crashing into skips outside my front door.

12.37 p.m. *Silent sailing ships*
Not bottle crashing skips

Do I feel inspired to write some verse?
No.

12.38 p.m. In my garden feeding the wildlife.
Breathing in the fresh chilly September air, and thinking of uplifting sea air.

12.40 p.m. Purrdita is lapping up some water in the kitchen. I'm daydreaming again about clear waters..... lapping on bracken-green-brown seaweed on the breakers..... and trying not to imagine the sound of clear, green and brown glass breaking.

3.41 p.m. Reading an article in Weekly Wife about Dawn French. There's a photograph of her most beautiful home by the sea, on the Cornish coast. Her front garden is the beach.

3.42 p.m. *Lucky Dawn.* There will be no bottles in her front garden. If there is one, it will be washed up on the sandy beach with the seaweed and shells. And there will be a message inside.

Thursday 16th

8.20 a.m. I can't lift the kettle.
Must remind Ben *again* not to fill it so full.

8.25 a.m. I can't get the song *Message in a bottle* out of my head.

8.35 a.m.	I don't want to wear my *bottle*-green hair scrunchie today. Groan. I was looking forward to an exciting change from the navy-blue scrunchie.
8.40 a.m.	Where *is* my navy-blue scrunchie? I can't find it *anywhere*.
9.15 a.m.	Still can't find navy-blue scrunchie. I am *not* going to wear bottle-green scrunchie. Will have to wear the bored-out-of-my-brain-brown one.
9.17 a.m.	Brown scrunchie is the colour of old beer bottles, will have to find my weary-grey or sleepy-blue scunchies with the floppy elastic.
9.20 a.m.	Wearing sleepy-blue, feeling floppy, and daydreaming of laying on my private sandy beach, the sound of the sleepy-blue sea lulling me to sleep.
9.21 a.m.	**CRASH! BANG! SMASH!**
	The builders next door are hammering and drilling. Two pictures have fallen off our sitting room wall. One picture is a sleeping fat ginger cat on a plump emerald green cushion. The other picture is a white tiger sleeping in the long jungle green grass.
9.23 a.m.	The glass in the frames has cracked.
9.24 a.m.	I'm imagining the ginger cat waking up, yawning, stretching, climbing out of the picture, and padding off to find a quieter place to sleep. The white tiger wakes up, growls, yawns, saunters out of the jungle grass, and out of the picture, then chases the ginger cat up the stairs.
9.25 a.m.	A black cat ornament has fallen off a shelf and the head has broken off. The ornament is a replica of the Egyptian goddess Bast, the goddess of love. She has fallen head over heels in love and completely lost her head.

9.26 a.m. Pick up body and head of cat ornament. I will glue them together, then see if I can find my thousand piece Egyptian pharaoh jigsaw puzzle, it will take my mind off *things*. Maybe if I fall off a shelf and my head breaks off, that *will* take my mind off things.

9.27 a.m. Need to find glue.

9.40 a.m. Find tube of UHU glue. The instructions tell you to coat both surfaces, then wait ten minutes.

9.41 a.m. Coat both surfaces.

9.51 a.m. The next part of the instructions brings to mind newly weds kissing (you press together briefly and vigorously, then an adjustment is no longer possible).

9.52 a.m. Press head on body briefly, with as much vigour as possible, then cat is like an engaged couple (stuck together, unless one of them decides to break things off, and finds themselves in a sticky situation, because it's *much* more difficult than they thought).

10.00 a.m. The goddess looks level headed and happier, in a serene Egyptian cat way.

10.02 a.m. I wish you could mend a broken heart with a little tube of glue. A tube of Cadbury's chocolate would help though; whenever someone at work was broken hearted or bereaved, I would give them chocolate. Hazelnut Twirls and After Eights were appreciated.

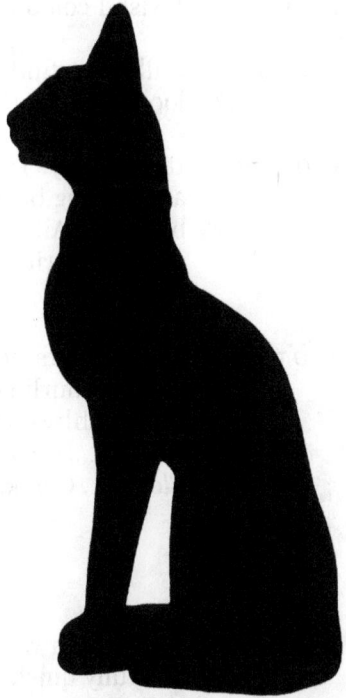

10.30 a.m.   I wish I could find my Egyptian jigsaw puzzle.

10.40 a.m.   Still can't find puzzle, and have worn myself out. Will look for it another day. I'm having one of *those* days.

11.05 a.m.   It's bin day. The bin men, wearing dirty yellow jackets, are hurling bulging black plastic sacks into a grimy grey bin lorry. All I'm aware of is the sound of breaking glass, and wondering what the future holds for our quiet little street.

3.10 p.m.   The builders next door, wearing dusty old check shirts, are now hurling dusty-pink-brown bricks and glass into the grubby old skip outside. *Smash..... **BANG***..... *CRASH..... Swear...... Crash..... Curse..... SMASH..... Clonk..... Clank..... Clink........... more unclean language.*

* * * * * * *

5.30 p.m.   Relaxing in warm 'Essence of ocean' bath. Our street is blissfully quiet. The house is blissfully quiet. I feel serene as Bast (the goddess of love) in my peaceful-dove-soapy-solitude, cleansing my body, mind and soul.

5.31 p.m.   I just wish I could get the song *Message in a bottle*, out of my head.

5.32 p.m.   *Sending out an SOS..... Sending out an SOS..... Sending out an SOS..... Sending out an SOS.....*

5.33 p.m.   *I hope that someone gets my.....*
              I hope that someone gets my.....
              I hope that someone gets my.....

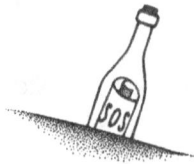

7.30 p.m.	*Coronation Street.*

7.30 p.m.   *Coronation Street.*
Steve gets a shock, not a message in a bottle, thank God. Kylie tries to buy his silence. Natasha desperately hopes she is pregnant, and Sean tells Owen what Liz *really* got up to.
Great! Lots of tears, *desperate* desperation, hopes and fears and a *big* shock. That will cheer up my evening!

Friday 17ᵗʰ

10.16 a.m.   In bath, rubbing Botanics aromatherapy massage oil into my fatigued shoulders. Relaxing..... calming..... soothing..... juniper berry, frankincense and orange.

10.20 a.m.   I'm feeling calm and relaxed, until I pick up a bottle of massage oil and a song pops into my head.....

I hope that someone gets my.....
I hope that someone gets my.....
I hope that someone gets my.....

***Massage** in a bottle*

11.35 a.m.   A Christmas gift catalogue arrives from the R.N.L.I.
I love to support the R.N.L.I., they once saved my friend Len's life at sea.

11.36 a.m.   Sometimes I feel all-at-sea.

11.37 a.m.   Ooh, little waves of verse are splashing into my mind.

My eyes
They are watering
I feel all-at-sea

I need the R.N.L.I.
To come and rescue me

11.45 a.m.   I think one day I will publish a book of some of my poems entitled, *Some of ME bad poetry.*

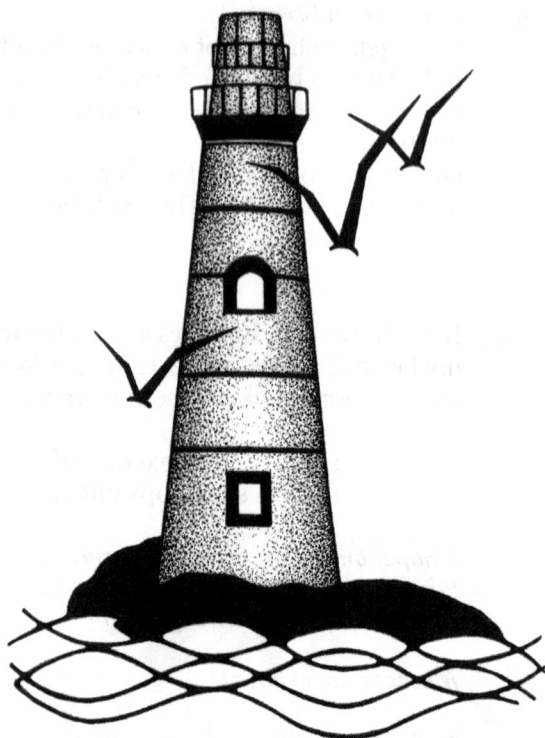

11.46 a.m.   Daydreaming about living by the sea again. I want my front garden to be the Cornish coast, maybe next door to Dawn French.

11.50 a.m.   Browsing through R.N.L.I. catalogue. Will order a couple of their calendars. Maybe the coastal calendar. Or shoreline flowers. The Little Corkers calendar looks cheerful; bright, colourful and amusing seaside paintings, by Nicky Corker.

11.51 a.m.   Tempted to order the sea urchin candle set or pebble lamp. They would look so perfect in my future home by the sea.

11.59 a.m.   The R.N.L.I. aims to reach casualties within ten nautical miles of lifeboat stations, within thirty minutes of launch in all weathers. They are so brave.

12.05 p.m.   I love their wall art. It would look brilliant on the walls of my home on the Cornish coast, next door to Dawn French.

12.06 p.m.   The wall art is hand crafted from hammered metal and lacquered for a distinctive lustrous finish. The catalogue says I will be delighted with how the new dimension wall art will transform and give new focus to a room, attracting interest and admiration. *Lovely!* The Regatta will look wonderful in the sitting room (on a seagull-grey wall) overlooking my private beach. The Lighthouse, on a sandy coloured wall in the bathroom. It will go nicely with my collection of seashells, jolly sailor light switch, seahorse and mermaid wall art, seaside postcards, tiny wooden beach huts, miniature wooden seagulls, white penguin shaped candle, sky-blue pillar candle (essence of seashore), pottery seals, photos of wild seals (taken at Seal Point on the Norfolk Coast), watercolours of whales and dolphins and deckchairs, a driftwood mirror, photos of Whitstable beach at sunset (in seaside themed frames bought in craft shops in Whitstable), and a pair of wind-up sharks that swim around in the bath.

I could invite Dawn French round to admire my art collection. She has written a book, so maybe I'll send her an R.N.L.I. catalogue c/o her publisher. Then one day, when I move next door, and she pops round for a cuppa,

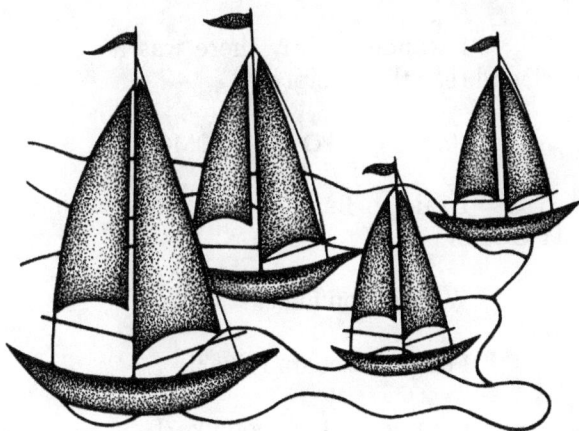

she'll say, 'Ooh! I've got the same one!' and we'll talk about how awful *and* wonderful it is to write a book. Then I'll read out my poem, Death by Chocolate, and we'll laugh a lot and eat too many chocolate seashells.

Saturday 18th

Ben took Cleopatra to our vet, Sally, for a flu injection and check-up. Getting a cat into a cat basket for a visit to the vet is not an easy job. Getting a stray cat into a cat basket and taking it to the vet, deserves a *big shiny medal*.

When Ben returned home he said, 'Cats like to ride on broomsticks don't they, can you take Cleopatra to the vet next time?!'

I replied, with my best witchy cackle, 'OK, but I'll need a bar of Galaxy Bubbles to give me a bit of extra lift, maybe two bars if the weather is bad.'

After a recovery-from-vet-visit-coffee and sugary snack, Ben drove into town to pick up a few things from Sainsbury's (mostly cat food) and Holland & Barrett (mostly my supplements). I comforted a disgruntled *I'm-never-going-to-the-vet-again* Cleopatra, and gave her a recovery-from-vet-gourmet-ocean-fish treat.

When Ben returned home later with carrier bags, I checked the Holland & Barrett till receipt, to see how much my oil of primrose oil capsules cost these days. The receipt read:

H&B   EPO   1000MG!   3.34

I wondered why there was an exclamation mark after 1000MG, and read the receipt as:

H&B   EPO   100 OMG!   3.34

I said to Ben, 'My primrose capsules are one hundred OH MY GODS!'

BEN: Wot are you like?!

ME: I dunno, wot am I like?!

BEN: I dunno, wot are you like?!

ME: I DUNNO!!

BEN: You've been overdosing on that Catherine Tate DVD again.

ME: *I KNOW! WOT AM I LIKE?!*

BEN: I DUNNO!

Purrdita looked up from her warm furry repose, and stared at us with a WHAT ARE THEY LIKE expression, then returned to sleepy feline dreamland.

7.30 p.m.   Hurrah! Have found Pharaoh jigsaw puzzle.

7.46 p.m.   Fed up now, can't find the tip of Tutankhamun's nose.

7.47 p.m.   Or the weird bird statue's eye.

7.56 p.m.   If I pick up one more piece of jigsaw puzzle that is lapis lazuli blue, a shade of gold, palm leaf green, or a hieroglyph, I'll *scream*.

7.58 p.m.   Will watch programmes about Pharaohs instead. Much more educational, less frustrating and mind numbingly boring. I can fall asleep if I want to, halfway through, with Cleopatra purring on my lap.

7.59 p.m.   Coping with M.E. can be like trying to do a million piece jigsaw, with endless sky-blue-sky and sandy-yellow-sand. Maybe a few palm trees, if you are lucky.

8.00 p.m.   *Ancient Egypt* : Documentary investigating how the architecture and engineering feats of Pharaohs Khufu and Ramesses the second, secured the Egyptian empire's place in history.

9.00 p.m.   *Tutankhamun: The Mystery Revealed.*
Documentary exploring the Egyptian Pharaoh's early years, looking at the story of his parents and their fate, the boy king's accession to the throne, and the many ways in which he transformed Egypt.

9.25 p.m.   I fell asleep, but woke up very inspired. I said to Ben, 'Hey, listen to this; Cleopatra, Cleopatra, on my lap you lazy lie, my lapis lazuli.' He nodded and gave me one of his *yes-yes-very-amusing-dear* looks.

Sunday 19th

Ben typed a letter to the waste reduction officer at our borough council offices, complaining about the proposed recycling site (proposed rubbish tip in our front garden).

He printed out thirty-five copies. Then printed the borough council's address on thirty-five envelopes. I stuck thirty-five turquoise stamps onto coffee brown envelopes. It was like Christmas without *Seasons Greetings,* festive Wallace and Gromit stamps on white envelopes, nativity scenes, jolly Santas, snowy scenes and glitter. I was tempted to change the words 'waste reduction' to 'waist reduction'. Ben posted the letters through the letter boxes of our neighbours, and the houses in the adjacent street, before I could do the wicked deed.

We hoped as many people as possible would sign the letters and post them. When Ben was posting a letter through the door of next-door-but-one, the door opened. Rose said how horrified she was at the proposals, and if Ben typed out a petition she would knock on all the doors. Ben said she wouldn't need to do anything, he'd sort it out. I *love it* when he's masterful.

Rose is very tiny, frail, white haired, and must be in her eighties. Her garden is picture-postcard-of-a-Cornish-cottage immaculate. Lots of roses. Vintage-wine-red, old-lady-hair-white, and grandmother's-lipstick-pink.

Half an hour after Ben had returned home from being a postman, Rose's neighbour knocked on our front door. I heard a beautiful Scottish male voice boom, 'Och aye, I'll be postin' ma letter on Monday an I'll be postin' yours too laddie!'

Monday 20th

9.08 a.m.   A pair of sycamore seeds flutter onto the bird table as I feed the wildlife. They remind me of a wishbone, so I make a wish – *please don't let the borough council turn our little street into a rubbish tip.*

11.25 a.m.   A parcel, booklet from BBC Audiobooks, two pamphlets, a Christmas gift catalogue, and a few letters are waiting for me, sprawled on the mat by the front door.

The post is sprawled on the mat. Not me. Only on a very bad day.

11.26 a.m.   Quite an exciting collection of post today. One of the letters has N.H.S. printed on the envelope. This doesn't usually mean good news so I will open it last.

11.27 a.m.   The N.H.S. letter is whispering meaningfully, 'You've got to open me sometime you know, it's important news, so you may as well get it over with girl.'
The parcel is shouting joyfully, 'Open me now! Open me first! You'll find lovely things to brighten your morning.'

11.28 a.m.   The pamphlets are for Super Pizza delivery and Thornton's Chocolates. I will not put my reading glasses on, so the photos of succulent mouth watering slices of pizza, and luscious, scrumptious looking chocolates, are all blurry.

11.29 a.m.   Put on reading glasses and peer into freezer. Hurrah! We have a Ristorante pizza; richly topped with tomatoes, mozzarella cheese and basil, on a crispy base.

11.30 a.m.   Text Ben:

CAN U PUT CHOC ON SHOPIN LIST – THANX X

11.32 a.m.   Ben replies:

WILL DO X

I love a man who is masterful *and* brings me chocolate.

11.33 a.m.   The booklet from the BBC Audio books collection looks interesting. I can't imagine life without my audio books now. I have all the Harry Potter audio books and Terry Pratchett's discworld series. I'm slowly adding to the collection.

11.34 a.m.   I think I may order *A Christmas Carol*, by Charles Dickens, read by Miriam Margolyes, for myself and an audio book loving friend. The CD will make a perfect Christmassy gift, and I like the drawings of Dickensian-type-characters-in-the-snow, on the cover of the case.

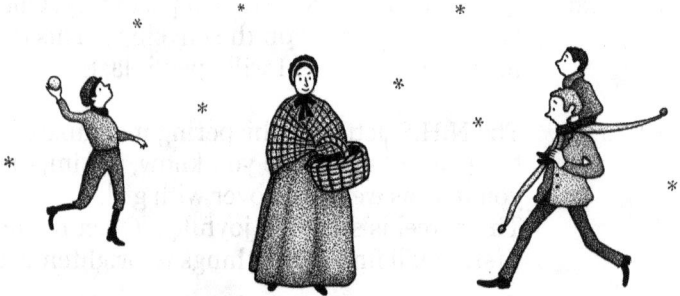

11.35 a.m.   I recall being part of the Dickens Festival, in Rochester, once upon a summertime in the early nineties. I was in the parade, dressed as a serving wench, with my friend's two teenage daughters, who were also dressed as wenches. We all had long hair, wore mop-caps, and really looked *the part*. Before the parade, we were standing around nearby a group of posh young ladies, dressed in beautiful nineteenth century costumes. They wore flouncy, lace and satin, pastel coloured dresses; frilly bonnets and curls, parasols and upper-class airs and graces. They all turned to stare at us, looking haughtily down their perfectly pink powdered noses, at the dirty common wenches. My young companions glared back angrily, but I was *most amused*; because for a moment, I felt transported back to the mid-eighteen hundreds and imagined a similar scenario in Rochester, all those decades ago, in Charles Dickens' day.

11.36 a.m.   I think he must have loved cats as much as I do. One of my favourite quotes was written by him.

What greater gift than the love of a cat?

CHARLES DICKENS

11.37 a.m.   *The Widows of Eastwick*, by John Updike, looks intriguing. I really enjoyed the film, *The Witches of Eastwick*, so I'm tempted to order that too.....

When the three witches – now old, remarried and widowed – go back to Eastwick to spend summer together, many things have changed. Darryl Van Horne is gone. But a chemistry still crackles between the three, and magic still lingers in the Eastwick air.

11.38 a.m.   The old witches in my book have fun doing spells to find a toy boy.....

That Cronella-crow-foot is after a toy boy again. There's going to be a lot of chanting to the God and Goddess, lighting of pink candles in rose quartz candle holders, and dancing on pink rose petals with no clothes on. At her age, honestly!

I don't feel the need to add, or change anything in my book about the old witches. I'm still making progress on the, I've-just-done-a-book front.

11.39 a.m.   Open parcel. It's the Christmas cards and paper from A.F.M.E. Great! Good variety of designs. I feel uplifted and a little Christmassy now.

11.42 a.m.   Leaf through Christmas gift catalogue from the Cancer Research charity. Will order the hot water bottle with

knitted cover, for a friend who is bed-ridden with M.E. - it's marshmallow pink with little cerise pink hearts.
The Cheer-up-your-cheese chutneys look ideal for Ben.
The Cosy-toes-Fair-Isle style socks, just right for me.
I'm tempted to order the Alan Titchmarsh watering can radio for auntie and uncle, to match the Alan Titchmarsh calendar I've ordered for them.

1.15 p.m.   Text message from Jayne:

> HI, I'VE BEEN TOTALLY POOPED – I HAD SOME BAD NEWS OVER THE WEEKEND – MY FRIEND DAVE WHO SPENT 8 YRS IN A BED BECOZ OF ME, HAD ALL BUT RECOVERED – I JUST SPOKE TO HIM WEEKS AGO – HE WAS TELLING ME NOT TO OVERDO IT – WELL, HE HAS HAD A HEART ATTACK – IS NOW BACK IN BED AS HE-S HAD A MAJOR RELAPSE – IT-S BEEN A REALITY CHECK FOR ME TO SLOW DOWN – TAKE IT EASIER – HOW R U? BIG WARM HUGS X X X

I feel so sad for Jayne's friend Dave. Will text her soon, when my hands aren't so achy.

6.05 p.m.   A neighbour, Pauline, who lives at the end of our street, No. 1, knocked on our door. She told Ben she had taken a petition round, opposing the recycling site, and had lots of signatures. She had also rung the borough council, but the waste reduction officer was away on holiday. How *very convenient*.

8.00 p.m.   Decide to open letter from N.H.S.
I'm invited to a routine breast cancer screening at our local hospital. I've had better invitations.
Need chocolate.

8.05 p.m.   My head is in the fridge, searching for a long dark green box with an ornate gold clock on the lid, the hands pointing to five past eight.

8.06 p.m.   As I remove the thin cellophane wrapper, a wonderful fresh minty fragrance caresses my nose. I reverently lift the box to my eager nostrils. I breathe in *very* deeply. I smile. I tingle. I'm so tempted. I carefully lift the lid. Delightful little black pockets of luxury await my indulgence. I stare in wonder.

8.07 p.m.   I pick a little pocket out of the middle. Maybe I'll take two. You've got to pick a pocket or two. Or three. Maybe I'll take the box to bed and eat the lot. I feel decadent. So naughty. Each delicate black pocket will have a gold clock printed on it, especially for me, telling me it's time to indulge. Within each pocket will be a darkly, deliciously, divinely thin square of cold crispy heaven. One side flat, the words *after eight* engraved many times. The other side with ripples, like a sandy beach when the tide is out. I so love darkness, a velvety texture, and sandy beaches on a Cornish coast.

8.08 p.m.   The witch in my book, loves velvety dark praline chocolates with a whole roasted hazelnut, because witches are often nutty and like to hide inside a dark velvety cloak. I was enjoying a box of Terry's All Gold, when I wrote that sentence; a much welcome birthday gift.
Writing is *so hard* when you are fatigued with M.E., and chocolate, especially plain chocolate, helps blood flow to the brain, giving you magical mental energy, memory and concentration. I cannot write, edit, or proofread without it.

8.09 p.m.   Nibble.... Nibble.... Nibble.... Nibble....
The sensually soft, sweet and creamy white centre is marvellously-minty-magical, melting on my tongue, and filling me with pleasure. I'm in chocolate nirvana.

8.10 p.m.   I offer the box to Ben and he comments, 'You love these don't you.'

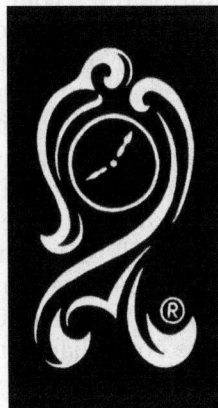

I reply casually, 'Yeah, they're OK.'
Then softly, mintily, cackle.

Tuesday 21ˢᵗ

La Redoute catalogue shot through the letterbox this
morning. The model on the cover was wearing this seasons military-
style coat, with double buttons, fine top-stitching, two patch pockets
with flaps *and* shoulder tabs. To add to the excitement, a lightweight
trench coat was mine for *FREE* with any order. The coat is double-
breasted with a big turn-up collar to flatter the neckline, and the
military inspired detailing is one of this season's *biggest* trends. Also
khaki is this season's *key* colour. How lovely.

When I flicked through the pages of TV Easy magazine,
I noticed there were lots of programmes about war this week, mostly
to mark the 70ᵗʰ anniversary of the Battle of Britain..... *First Light*: A
one-off drama based on personal memoirs of Geoffrey Wellum, an
R.A.F. Pilot who fought in the Battle of Britain with the legendary 92
Squadron..... *Words of the Blitz*: Diaries and letters of people affected
by the Blitz.

As I sat in the kitchen, waiting for the kettle to come to
the boil for my afternoon cuppa, I watched the second hand marching
relentlessly, perfectly precisely, past black numbers on the large white
face of the kitchen clock. I recalled the days I relentlessly marched off to
school, sometimes avoiding the cracks in the precisely placed paving
slabs of the pathways. I woke up every morning to the sound of a very
loud ominous siren, at precisely eight o'clock. It was originally used
during the second world war, to warn civilians of an impending air-
raid; fire bombs would be falling from enemy planes onto our precious
homes. Now it warned workers at a nearby factory, every weekday
morning, that it was time to start work.

We lived next door to a big old house used as a youth
club. I spent many youthful evenings there playing table tennis, or
sitting chatting with friends in the window seats of the big old bay
windows. We were forbidden to use an ouija board, because the house
was built on an ancient burial mound. This meant the grounds were
about eight feet higher than our garden, and an ivy covered bank,
topped with tall bushes, separated our garden from the small estate.
The house had survived the second world war, you could see where

the fire bombs had fallen through the roof. One bomb still lay, quietly, hiding in the ivy covered bank.

During my childhood; nearby where my brother, sister and I splashed about in our buttercup yellow paddling pool, there lurked a sinister snake in the grass. But it wasn't a snake. And it wasn't in the grass. A German fire bomb silently dozed with one menacing eye open, watching us from beneath an ivy-green quilt; close to where mum tended her British red roses, hung out white sheets from British Home Stores to dry on the washing line, kept the pegs in a navy blue peg-bag, and dad snoozed in a Union Jack deck chair with a knotted hankie on his head.

The menacing eye, blinking like a patient predator, must have been gritty with rust, because the bomb had lain hidden for almost thirty years before it was finally discovered. By dad. Hundreds of snails and slugs must have slithered over it, worms wormed under it, and creepy crawlies scuttled past it, thinking it was just an innocent lump of metal. Maybe they could hear a faint ticking sound.

One Saturday afternoon, when I was in my teens, I returned home from a shopping trip in town and was surprised to see an army truck parked outside our house. Dad had been digging in the ivy bank, removing the ivy so he could plant creepers, when he found something long and metal. He usually found grey slow worms, and held them up to me so I could stroke them on the head, and say hello. On this occasion, the three inch thick and fifteen inch long grey thing was not to be held up to a little girl, so she could gently pat it on the head, and say hello. The nice soldiers took the incendiary bomb away.

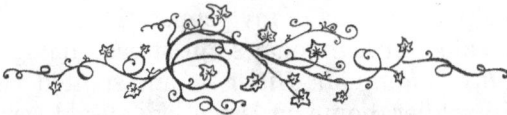

Sipping my afternoon tea, I recalled the days I sat sketching at Chatham dockyard, when I attended the art college at Fort Pitt, Rochester, in the seventies. Dad said he had to run up and down the steep banks of Fort Pitt with a rucksack on his back, in his army training days. My first day at college, I was asked to bring an object to draw. I brought one of my dad's army boots.

I used to love visiting the dockyard, sketching or painting miniature watercolours. Sometimes a dear old war veteran would sit beside me and tell me his wartime stories. Some of them were *so sad*. One day a tear rolled down my cheek, and dripped onto the sketchpad resting on my lap. It mingled with the khaki and camouflage green waters of my painting of the river Medway. Then it started to spit with rain, but the effect on my painting was *really good*. The old war veteran and young art student laughed.

* * * * * *

The second hand of the kitchen clock marched on as I continued to sip my peppermint tea. It looked ivy-green (the tea, not the second hand). I stared at the big white face of the kitchen clock and yawned a big wide yawn. Almost two o'clock. I considered turning on the TV to watch an afternoon film and take my mind off sad memories. The TV magazine lay open on the coffee table, showing Tuesday's viewing. I noticed today's entertaining films were: *Appointment in London*, a World War Two drama starring Dirk Bogarde; *Sea of Sand*, a World War Two adventure starring Richard Attenborough; and *Battle of the Bulge*, starring Henry Fonda. I had a book once, written by his daughter Jane Fonda, about diet and exercise – battling with 'the bulge'.

I wouldn't have minded watching an episode of the hilarious comedy, *Dad's Army*; starring Arthur Lowe (Captain Mainwaring, commander of the Walmington-on-Sea Home Guard) John Le Mesurier (Sergeant Wilson) and the rest of Dad's Army: Lance Corporal Jones, Private James Frazer, Private Joe Walker, Private Charles Godfrey and the young lad, Private Frank Pike. I always sang along to the theme when the series was on, and knew *all* the words.

I sipped the last of my peppermint tea and sang quietly to myself, as I leafed through today's Christmas catalogue..... '*Who do you think you are kidding Mr. Hitler*.....' and spotted a gift that made me smile like a soldier, home on leave; like an old war veteran who finds friendship with a young artist at Chatham dockyard; like a little girl stroking the head of a grass snake. I decided to order the gift for a friend who, like me, loves boiled eggs for breakfast, and dunking hot buttery toast soldiers into warm creamy egg yolk. There were many times I noticed a tell-tale yellow blot on his check shirt.

I met the late Spike Milligan once upon a lunchtime in the eighties, at a book signing in Waterstones, Maidstone. I couldn't help noticing a dribble of egg yolk on his red and blue tie; a colourful compliment to his wonderful eccentric humour, and what a *charmingly lovely* man. One of my comedy heroes. He signed my copy of his book, *Adolf Hitler: my part in his downfall*, with beautiful large curly black writing and we exchanged witty banter, making each other laugh *a lot*. I was most thrilled and flattered, all the way up to my fluttering Maybelline eyelashes, chocolate mousse coloured eyelids and neatly plucked eyebrows. I floated all the way back to work with a big grin on my face.

I have digressed, and now return to the subject of the Christmas gift I decided to order for the boiled-egg-and-toast-loving-friend. It's an egg cup. A soldier egg cup. The egg cosy is a black soldier's hat which sits neatly on the cup; a little face wearing a red regimental jacket and black boots. He is holding a small red plastic spoon. The egg cup and cosy comes in a gift box with a toast cutter, and the cutting-out-bits are the shape of soldiers standing to attention. It's one of those gifts *I know* I'll be tempted to keep for myself, because it makes me laugh *and* I collect egg cups. *AND* laughter is the best medicine to take with your boiled egg and toast soldiers in the morning.

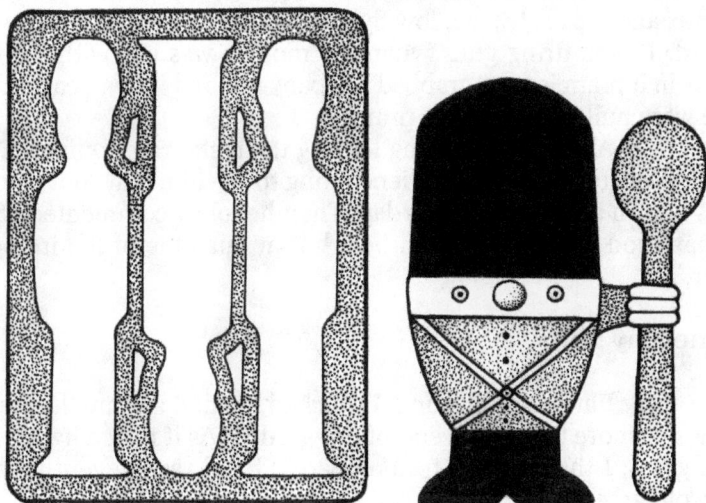

I recall one summer's day, when I had an appointment with my osteopath, I saw a middle-aged man, driving a bright red shiny sports car with an open top, park outside the clinic. He had a rather large, bald, egg shaped head. Sitting low in the driver's seat, he brought to mind a boiled egg, sitting in a bright red shiny egg cup.

I told my osteopath about the sporty-egg-head, thinking it would *crack* her up. That she would be *most* amused. She didn't laugh, just managed a half smile, and I wondered if he were a friend or relative. Maybe an uncle.

When my appointment was over, I spotted the egg-head (my osteopath's latest boyfriend) sitting in the waiting room. As I settled into a nearby chair to wait for my taxi, I was *very* tempted to ask him lots of questions. Was he *free range* and free to roam in the daytime? Did he have a *Lion quality* tattoo, to show he had been laid in the UK? Was he about to get laid again? What size was he, a medium or a large? How were things going with my osteopath, did he sometimes feel a little hen pecked? Was she helping him come out of his shell? Had she cracked it?

Just before eleven tonight, Ben returned home from his gig at the Mexxa Mexxa restaurant, and said there's a dear old man, David, who comes to see his duo play. He told Ben he remembers the Blitz, and his family had to move three times. He was a little boy at the time, and recalls when a low flying plane flew over the street where he lived. It was firing guns when his mother was out with his baby brother in a pram, so she grabbed the baby and ran into a nearby alley. There were bullet holes in the pram.

As Ben was leaving leaving the restaurant tonight, David said he'd like to bring his girlfriend along to see him play, but she only comes out on a Friday or Saturday. Then he jokily commented, 'She's not that good at cooking, or in bed, but at our time of life it doesn't matter.'

Wednesday 22nd

Early this morning, I watched my first autumn leaf falling from a sycamore tree at the end of our garden. As it rested lightly on a tuft of grass, I thought of a frail old lady's hand resting gently on her lumpy old green quilt.

In the grounds behind our garden there is an old people's home. The rooftops of the building are almost at eye level when I look out of the kitchen window, because there's a twenty-something foot drop at the end of our garden. During winter months, I often watch the sun setting behind a silhouette of bare sycamore tree branches,

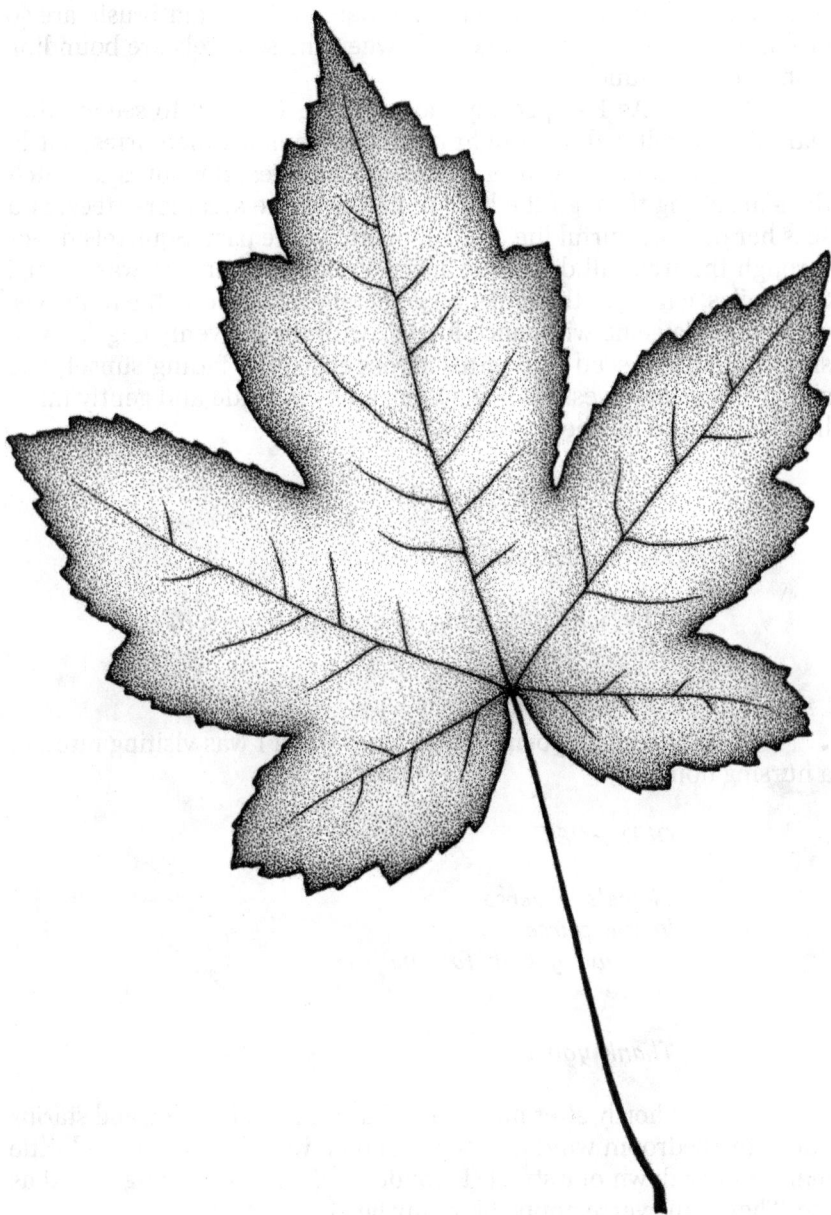

ornate rooftops and chimney pots. Crimson, purply-pinks and golds, softly blended together with a cosmic water-colour paintbrush, are so enchanting and peaceful; especially when the squirrels are bounding along the tree branches.

As I sipped my morning tea, I waited to see another leaf fall and felt sad. I thought of an old woman's memories, softly fading away like the steam from my morning tea. She loves to watch the sun setting through the bare branches of the sycamore trees, and sees her once colourful life as a silhouette of the past. Squirrels dance through the trees all day. Ruth loved to dance when she was young. She smiles, gazing at the pink and golden beauty beyond the branches, where one day, she will dance forever with the heavenly angels. As a single sycamore seed pirouettes across the softly fading sunset, she slowly closes her eyes. An angel appears by her side and gently takes her by the hand for the last dance.

Now, I've made myself cry.

Tears are streaming down my face.

Why, *why why why,* do I do this to myself.

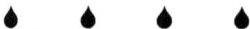

♦　♦　♦　♦

I recall a poem I wrote once when I was visiting mum in a nursing home.

OLD POET

There's a verse
In me purse
Can you get it for me
Nurse

Thank you dear

Shortly after mum passed away, I recall sitting and staring out of the bedroom window one afternoon, watching a thin, sad little man wander down our street. I wondered if he were feeling as sad as me. Then some verse popped into my head.

TIME

Time held me
By the hand
And told me
Not to cry

There's always
A tomorrow
And the man
Walked by

The kitchen clock, tick..... tock..... ticked another weary Wednesday morning away. The cold tap, drip..... drop..... dripped my weary life away. I needed a little piece of heavenly chocolate.

I wondered if it was OK to eat *After Eight* mints after 8 a.m., for an early morning treat. It didn't take me long to decide. After only one tick of the clock and one drip of the tap, I knew it was perfectly-peppermintly fine to indulge oneself in a little luxury first thing. An *excellent* idea. My spirits lifted after two delicious squares of cold crispy delight. My sadness drifted away above the sycamore trees, to sail away with the clouds in a sleepy-ocean-blue sky..... a fluffy turtle cloud became a Canada goose..... a seahorse head grew a long snout..... an octopus with five legs chased a leaping frog.

The peace of my day was broken in the afternoon. Shattered, like the glass in my pictures that fell off the wall, when the builders were busy next door. Cracked, like the shell of my egg, when I took it out of the fridge and boiled it; the escaping egg white, a tiny fluffy cloud. Loud voices filled the car park. Shrill, excited, full-of-youth-and-life voices. Endless chatter. Exuberant laughter.

I peered out of the sitting room window, to see several groups of little boys wearing bottle green sweat-shirts and grey back-to-school trousers, wandering across the car park, on their way home from school. I started to feel grey. My mind filled with dull rainy day thoughts, and all I could think of was the sound of smashing green bottles. Brown bottles and clear glass bottles, crashing into recycling skips. I needed more chocolate.

After three squares of minty heaven, bright happy sunny thoughts filled my mind. I could hurl our empty bottles out of the bedroom window, aiming for the recycling skips! It could be my *new hobby*. I may, accidentally-on-purpose, hit the waste reduction officer on the head as she throws away her wine bottles. She will have a lot of bottles because she must be an alcoholic, a little insane or something, to consider installing five recycling skips so close to houses *and* an old people's home.

Early evening, I heard my new neighbour open his front door, and plonk two black bin liners full of rubbish on the path, ready for the bin men to collect tomorrow morning. I was acutely aware of the sound of clanking glass, and wondered if maybe he would like to join me in my *new hobby*.

Life isn't too bad really. After all, we've got kitchen roll with a new design, a delightful change from the usual herbs or flowers. Very colourful. Lots of greens. Very designery. Unfortunately I cannot feel overjoyed, or delighted. It's a bottle design. But Weekly Wife is quite exciting this week; Wendy tells me to mix stylish prints with dramatic colour for a sophisticated and sexy look, without being too girly or fussy. Some of the bold flower and leaf prints are tasteful, not a bottle design in sight.

Wendy suggested I try some wall art too; the Fleur de Lys stencil from Henny Donovan's new damask range will create a truly individual look, and it works equally well on white or coloured backgrounds. I had to admit I liked the idea, and red on a white background *did* look dramatic and *truly individual*, but all I can manage these days is a splash of tomato soup on the kitchen wall. That will have to do for now.

I'm not very enamoured by Wendy's choice of vase. It's the most horrible *hideous* vase I've ever seen, almost as ugly as my ex-husband. The glaze is aqua haze bullet crackle and it's very near bullet shaped, like his head was. Is the vase supposed to match this season's military-style-fashion?

Wendy's top tip for the week, is to paint the wall behind my bed with a bold colour, it could transform my bedroom in a weekend. This is *truly wonderful* to know.

8.00 p.m.   Feel like shooting myself.

8.01 p.m.   Time for more minty squares of delight.

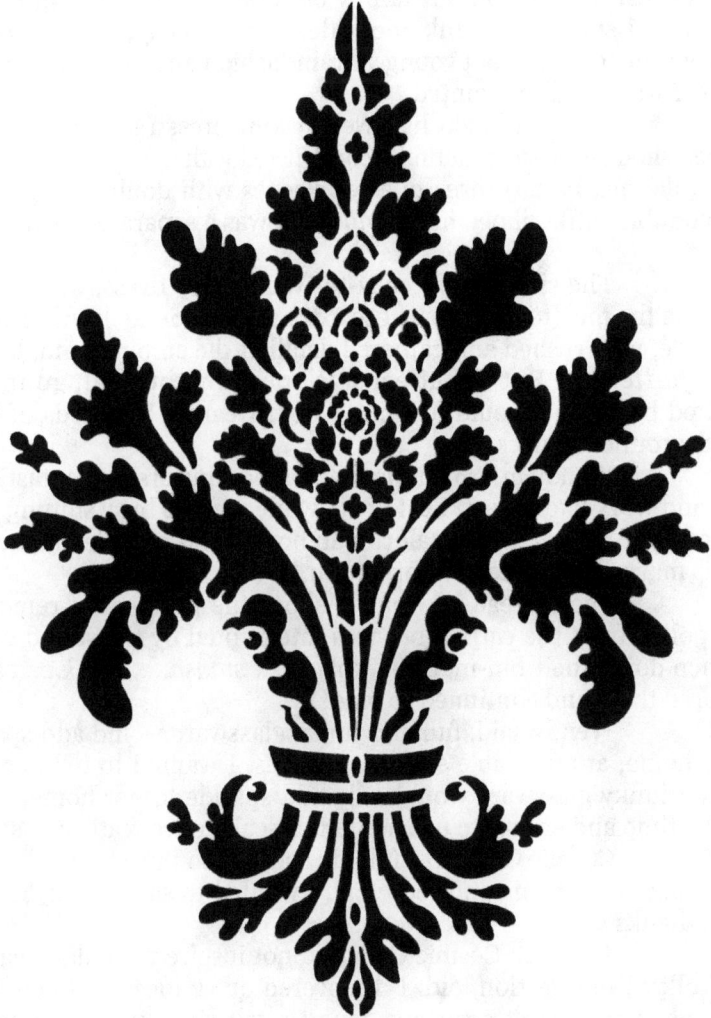

Thursday 23rd

As I watched three autumn leaves flutter down..... down..... down to rest in peace on our lumpy old lawn, I couldn't help feeling sad again. I started to think about death and decay, so I picked up Weekly Wife to read about young vibrant fashion and up-to-the-minute advice. I was not disappointed.

The soft-khaki lightweight knit dress (good if you have fatigued shoulders) was beautifully constructed with a fine rib contrasting waist (like me, ha ha) three-quarter sleeves with double rough cuffs and a double ruffle ribbed hem, *and* there was a separate jersey under slip.

The simple-and-easy-to-wear jersey dress, with a little stretch in the mix (to allow for those extra winter pounds) a fixed cross-over style, with ruched and gathered detail at the empire seam, looked *super flattering*. But the effect was spoilt by the oval, gunmetal coloured beading; I would feel like I were wearing hundreds of little bullets around my neck.

Wendy informed me that feather dusters are fantastically retro and work like a treat. Best of all, while you are busy shining your surfaces, you'll burn up 173 calories an hour. I was completely thrilled by this marvellous piece of information.

Then I read in wonder about the problem of removing shoe polish from the carpet, but was interrupted by the sound of the bin men doing their bin-men-job. *Crash..... smash..... clank..... clonk.* I ignored them and continued to read.

Wendy said, fun and funky glassware would add sparkle to my home, at affordable smashing prices. I wanted to tell her that fun and funky glassware would only add sparkle to her home, if she had the time and energy to use her fantastically retro feather duster.

Cosmic Colin was full of wisdom too this week, about re-evaluating, re-thinking and recycling. I wanted to say to him, 'Cheers Colin, thanks *a lot*'.

Although Cosmic Colin did not inspire me today, reading the Trolley Dolly section, did. I discovered quick ideas and new buys from the supermarket spy, then found a felt tip pen, and drew the trolley dolly hurling bottles into her trolley.

I felt *much* better.

Friday 24th

1.10 p.m. HURRAH! Thirty copies of my book, *Love & Best Witches*, arrive from Epic Press. Shiny and new. Magical, purpley-midnight-blue.

2.35 p.m. GREAT! Thirty jiffy bags arrive from e-bay. Crisp and clean. White as flour. Airkraft bags, light as puff pastry.

2.36 p.m. CACKLE! CACKLE! I have a wonderful wodge of witchy paper (printed out for me by Ben) ready for all the letters I need to write. I've decorated the paper with a border, to match the drawings in my witchy book, and made it colour-ful; pumpkin orange, scary scarlets, herbal greens, potion purples, magical magentas and spooky blues.

2.37 p.m. BRILLIANT! I have Berol italic pens, witchy-cauldron-black, and books of stamps, old-wizard-boots-brown.

6.00 p.m. PHEW! *Well done me.*

Twelve books beautifully parcelled up with letters (short letters) for friends, family and A.F.M.E. That's the first batch done, ready for Ben to take to the post office tomorrow. I will be too exhausted to move an eyelash tomorrow.

Saturday 25th

9.00 a.m. I'm not going to move much today.

9.01 a.m. Or think much.

11.35 a.m. My Goodwill Christmas catalogue arrives.

11.40 a.m. If I sit in the garden the wind will turn the pages for me.

11.50 a.m. Sitting in garden.

11.51 a.m. A kind breeze turns the pages for me.

11.53 a.m.   I like the cotton tea-towel with a black cat design, and lots of paw prints.

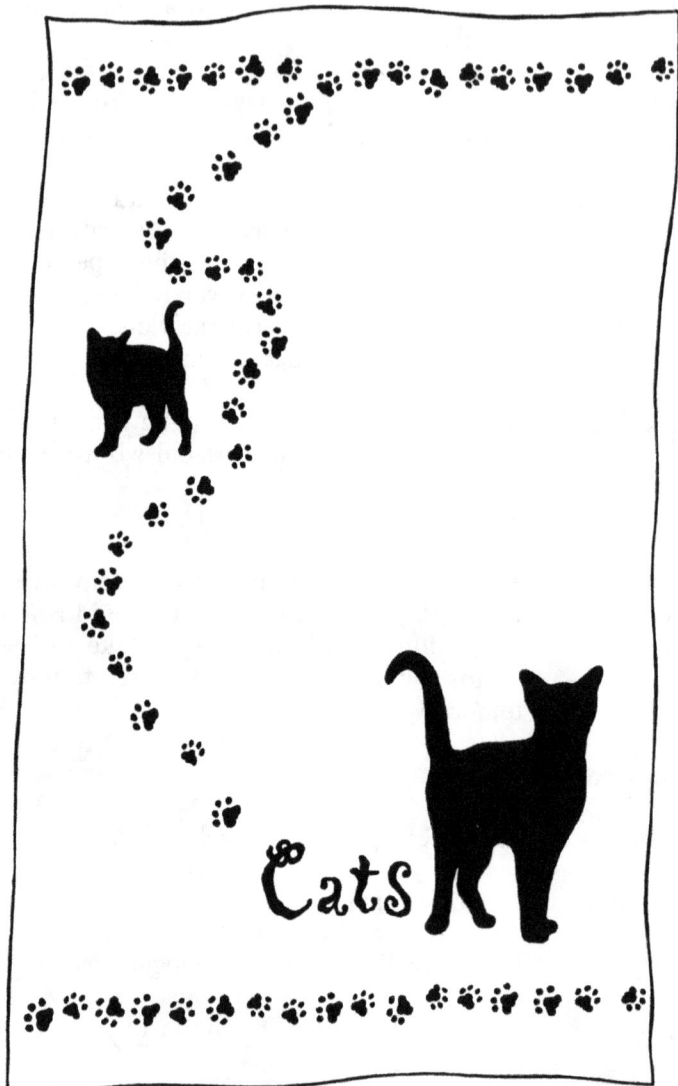

11.54 a.m.   I *do not* like the *bottle green* Rovers Return bottle bank: a drink in a bottle to celebrate 50 years of *Coronation Street*. There's a matching bottle opener and a slot in the bottle top, so you can collect spare change in the bottle if you wish. That's nice.

1.00 p.m.   In bath, rubbing Botanics aromatherapy massage oil into my right shoulder. Will find energy to massage left shoulder tomorrow.

1.01 p.m.   I'm comforted and soothed by sweet marjoram, ylang ylang and mandarin, but there's a song I can't get out of my head.

1.02 p.m.   *I hope that someone gets my.....*
             I hope that someone gets my.....
             I hope that someone gets my.....

             Massage in a bottle

Sunday 26th

10.00 a.m.   Long soak in warm Radox muscle-soak-bubble-bath, with clary sage and sea minerals.

10.02 a.m.   Daydreaming about my dream home by the sea, on the Cornish coast, next door to Dawn French.

10.03 a.m.   I wonder if she has ever found a message in a bottle on her beach-front-garden.

10.05 a.m.   I've got *that song* in my head *again*.

10.06 a.m.   So v. tired. So v. achy after Friday's efforts. Was it worth it? *Yes,* definitely.

10.08 a.m.   I'm looking forward to *Coronation Street*. Natasha is released from hospital and she's going to drop Gail in it. About time too. Naughty Gail revealed Natasha's private medical records.

Monday 27th

9.31 a.m.   Plod slowly into garden to feed the wildlife. It's getting very wintry now, my thin black dressing gown with pink paw print design, feels inadequate.

11.45 a.m.   Browsing through The Original Gift Company catalogue, that has just flown in through the letterbox. The melting clock (a homage to the surrealist Salvador Dali) will be a lovely gift for Dad, who admires the artist.

11.48 a.m.   Sometimes life seems surreal when you have M.E. Sometimes you sleep so much and have such vivid dreams, that reality and the dream world blur together in your foggy brain.

11.49 a.m.   Last summer I had a surreal moment that I recall vividly. Voices outside in our street, had woken me up early, and I peered out of the bedroom window. It was light, a pale misty blue morning, about 5.30 a.m. Four very tall, slim, young women, slowly appeared out of the mist. Lots of frothy, bright-candy-floss-pink hair tumbled to their waists. They looked like ballet dancers, wearing white tutu-type dresses, thick white tights and flat white ballet pumps. If they had been silent and staring they would have appeared a little sinister, like John Wyndham's Midwich Cuckoos; but they seemed rather sweet as they ambled along the path giggling, and sometimes stumbling off the kerb, into the road.
I watched them slowly disappear into the mist, wondering if they were some kind of comedy act. They wouldn't have been such a strange sight if it were early evening, but at daybreak, when you've just woken up with an M.E. foggy brain and it's misty.....
I plodded back to bed and had very weird, pink, white and blue dreams; then awoke late morning wondering if it had *all* been a dream.

11.55 a.m.   More catalogue browsing. I like the vintage-style wall-mounted wirework mannequin. Sometimes you feel like a wall-mounted mannequin when you have M.E. Stiff. Lifeless. All you do is hang around the house all day.

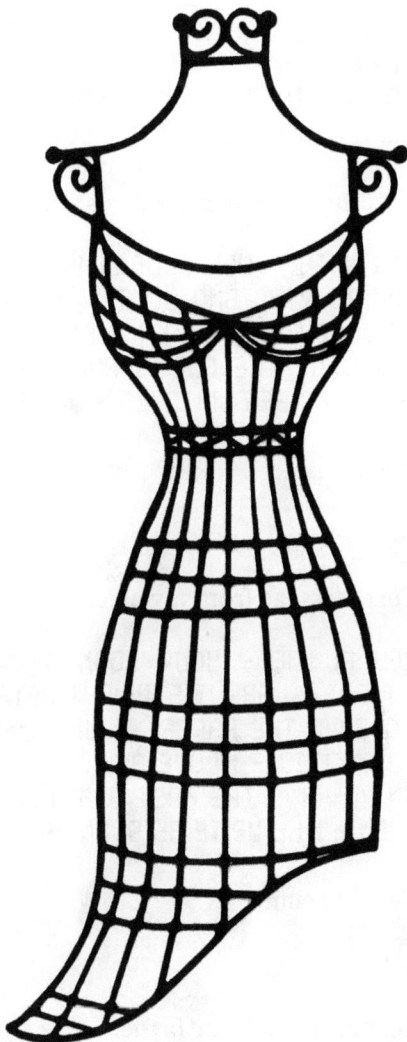

Tuesday 28th

11.40 a.m.   Text message from Jayne:

> OH WITCHY FRIEND – WHAT A WONDERFUL SURPRISE I
> JUST GOT IN THE POST – THE BOOK LOOKS GREAT – I
> WANTED TO TXT YOU 1ST – OFF TO READ IT NOW –
> WELL DONE – I CAN-T BELIEVE IT – WITCHY HUGS XXX

6.45 p.m.   Text message from Ben's sister:

> HI VERITY – WOW – BOOK IS FANTASTIC – IT-S SUCH
> FUN TO READ AND YOUR DRAWINGS ARE WONDERFUL –
> WE LOVE IT – AND I KNOW KIRA WILL TOO – THANKS SO
> MUCH FOR THE COPIES AND GLAD WE COULD HELP –
> LOVE AND BEST WITCHES – JULIA AND PAUL XXX

6.46 p.m.   Big Smile.

Wednesday 29th

8.03 a.m.   Text message from my niece:

> HEY AUNTIE – YOUR BOOK ARRIVED YESTERDAY – I
> LOVE IT – I SAW IT STRAIGHT AFTER SCHOOL AND WHEN
> I OPENED THE PARCEL IT WAS LIKE – AHHHHH – I WAS
> SO EXCITED – I LOVE ALL THE DRAWINGS – THE FAIRY
> ON PG 48 IS THE MOST BEAUTIFUL DRAWING I-VE EVER
> SEEN – I-LL WRITE AS SOON AS I CAN – PROMISE X

8.04 a.m.   Very big smile.

Thursday 30th

8.03 p.m.   Text message from Jayne:

> WITCHY FRIEND U R AMAZING – HOW ON EARTH DID U
> WRITE A BOOK LET ALONE ILLUSTRATE IT? I-M LOVING
> IT – THANK U FOR MAKING IT HAPPEN – HUGS XXX

8.04 p.m.   Huge pumpkin grin.

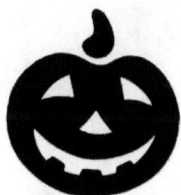

Chapter Two

October

Friday 1ˢᵗ

8.20 a.m.   HURRAH! I've survived nine months of *another* year,
coping with author anxiety, proposed-rubbish-tip anxiety,
M.E., myself, and *too many* bad hair days. *Well done me!*

11.45 a.m.   YIPEEE! Yellow Moon (the children's charity) Xmas
catalogue has arrived, full of fun, creative, card making
ideas for children. Excellent for grown-ups who are
housebound and unable to venture out to buy birthday
cards, Easter cards, Christmas cards..... Their party paper
plates, melamine cups, plates and bowls are beautifully
light for weak hands to pick up. The pink melamine plates
(I ordered last year) with cupcake, teapot and heart design
are delightful.

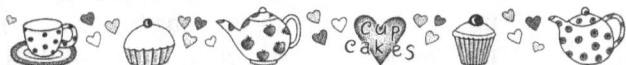

The face painting kits are perfect for when you want to
paint your face green, or cover your face with red spots,
so people will stop telling you *how well* you look.

11.46 a.m.   LOVELY! The Love Lavender Christmas gifts catalogue
has arrived too. I *love* their creamy lavender coloured hand
and body lotion, and it's such a healing fragrance. It helps
me to stay calm and peaceful, on days when I want to drown
myself in the bath. The Norfolk English lavender cologne
roll-on is great for days when your hands are too weak to
use a spray scent. I'm hoping Santa will give me Cotswold
Lavender bath salts and soap for Christmas. And maybe a
little jar of their soothing gel, with lavender and peppermint, it's really *cool.*

Love Lavender

2.13 p.m.   OH JOY! My Ravensburger puzzle has arrived. A Disney panoramic thousand piece jigsaw puzzle. I'm enjoying recognising all the colourful characters; Peter Pan and Tinkerbell, Alice in Wonderland, the Little Mermaid, Aladdin, Mickey Mouse, Snow White and the Seven Dwarves..... thousands of minutes of fun ahead. There seems to be a lot of yellow tiles and pillars, foliage and midnight blue sky in the background; reminding me of puzzles with too much sky, sea and sandy beach..... no, no, I will see it as an exciting new challenge. I will experience many moments of small achievement, when I finally find *that little piece of puzzle to complete that particular part of the picture*..... hours of looking forward to finally seeing *the BIGGER picture*. The big bright and beautiful picture.
I feel inspired to write a song about puzzles bright and beautiful, with creatures great and small; characters wise and wonderful, Walt Disney made them all. I could make up the verses, piecing the song together, as I join the puzzle pieces together. Maybe have lots of different melodies inspired by Disney tunes.....
I like some of the soft ice-cream colours, the raspberry pink stripes on the grinning Cheshire cat, and the golden toffee colours of Bambi and the Lion King..... Delicious days of *pure panoramic pleasure* ahead..... which tasty little piece of puzzle shall I choose next?
Can't wait.

6.06 p.m.   WONDERFUL! Pauline, from number one at the end of our street, has knocked on our door and given Ben a copy of the list of signatures she collected, opposing the proposed recycling site.

6.09 p.m.   BRILLIANT! I'm reading all the signatures with addresses, on two A4 sheets of paper. Big bold writing. Tiny, *slanting forwards* writing. Tall, slanting backwards writing. Very rounded confident letters. Written in capitals. Mad writing. Very wobbly writing. All very brilliant. Oh God. *Oh God, oh God, please don't let the borough council turn our peaceful little street into a noisy rubbish tip.*

Saturday 2nd

8.35 a.m.   OH, S**T! My frog prince pyjama bottoms feel a little damp.
Damp as a frog on a lily pad. Damp as the pillow of the
broken hearted. Damp as a love letter, the ink a little
smudged with tears. Not the whole of my pyjama bottoms.
Just the crotch area. Damn. I must remember not to sit
on the toilet (resting after brushing my teeth) when the
lid is *up* and my pyjama bottoms are *not down*. And I'm
in my usual (miles away) state of daydream. And I'm
re..... lax..... ed.

8.36 a.m.   I put pyjama bottoms in the washing machine. May as
well wash the top too, even though I've only worn it one
night. It was a sweaty-nightmarish-night. All bloomin'
night.

8.37 a.m.   I put myself in school detention, and mentally write out
three times; *I must not sit on the toilet when the lid is
up and I'm wearing p-j's.* Pee-j's, haha. Don't know why
I'm laughing. But you have to, don't you.

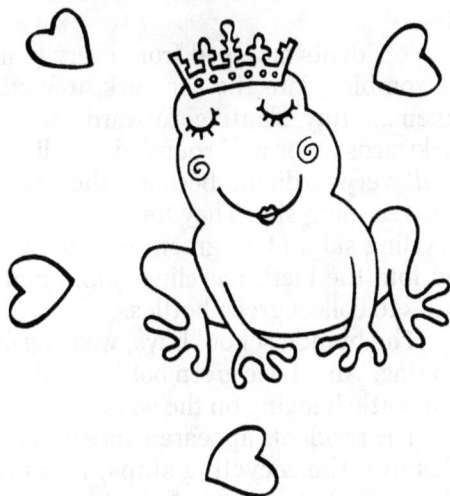

I felt exhausted all morning after the nightmares. Nothing unusual there, except they were more spookily sinister than I normally experience.

Ten little school boys wearing bottle green uniforms, stood statue still, solemnly staring into space, in the car park opposite our house. There was something eerie about their pale faces, bright green eyes and perfect, short blonde hair. I recalled John Wyndham's Midwich Cuckoos, and shivered.

I sat mesmerised, staring out of the window, watching the icy-cold-looking boys, from the warmth of my small bedroom. Then I shivered again as each one in turn, looked up at me, their bright green eyes boring into my soul. Their complexion, yellow and blue as cheddar cheese going mouldy. They *knew* I was opposed to the wonderful recycling site.

The boys started to sing, in a joyless manner, 'Ten green bottles hanging on the wall, ten green bottles hanging on the wall.....'

I froze with fear and the bottle-green hair scrunchie around my pony tail began to tighten. It grew *tighter* and *tighter* until all my hair fell out. My teeth ached, and fell out into the palms of my cupped hands. Every tooth had turned moss green. The school boys continued to sing, 'There'll be seven green bottles hanging on the wall.....' and pointed to the five new shiny black recycling skips in the car park. One for unwanted hair, one for teeth, the other three for green bottles.

Residents emerged from every house in our street. They walked like zombies, into the car park, towards the recycling skips. Big bold men..... tiny slanting forwards women..... some tall and slanting backwards..... or well rounded..... a little mad..... very old and wobbly..... *all* very brilliant because they had signed the petition opposing the recycling site. They tore out their hair and threw it into the hair recycling skip. Moss green teeth fell into cupped hands, and were hurled into the teeth recycling skip. Then they slowly returned to their homes to collect green bottles.

The blonde school boys, wearing-bottle green uniforms continued to sing, 'And if one green bottle should accidentally fall, there'll be one green bottle hanging on the wall.....'

The residents appeared once more in the car park, to hurl their bottles into the recycling skips. I was too afraid to venture out, so I threw my bottles out of the bedroom window. One of my bottles did accidentally fall, *accidentally-on-purpose,* onto the head of the waste reduction officer, who was throwing her empty wine bottles into a skip. It knocked her out. Cold. The school boys ended their song and began to march, crocodile fashion, out of the car park. On their way, they stepped over the body of the waste reduction officer without looking at her, as she lay motionless. Then they turned into a bottle-green crocodile, who ate the waste reduction officer. The creature burped, spat out her shoes, and smiled.

A nightmare with a happy ending, although I don't think my borough council would agree.

Almost everything was green in this week's Weekly Wife. In the Trolley Dolly treats section: an avocado green bra and shorts set from Diamond boutique at Tesco, an olive green rose ring, basil green ballet-type-shoes and tropical lime shower sorbet, from Asda. In the Home Trends section: green wine glasses from Tesco, an 'eat your greens' screen print from Beth Stevens, funky olive green table napkins from Dunhelm Mill, funky green star place mats and coasters from Funky Olive, and a leaf green, leaf design rug from Next.

I quite liked the leafy-green-leafy-design rug and avocado green underwear. I showed the photo of the bra and knickers to Ben, and asked him if he would be thrilled if I wore underwear to match the name of his duo. He pretended to show enthusiasm. I'm sure the diners at Mexxa Mexxa would be more

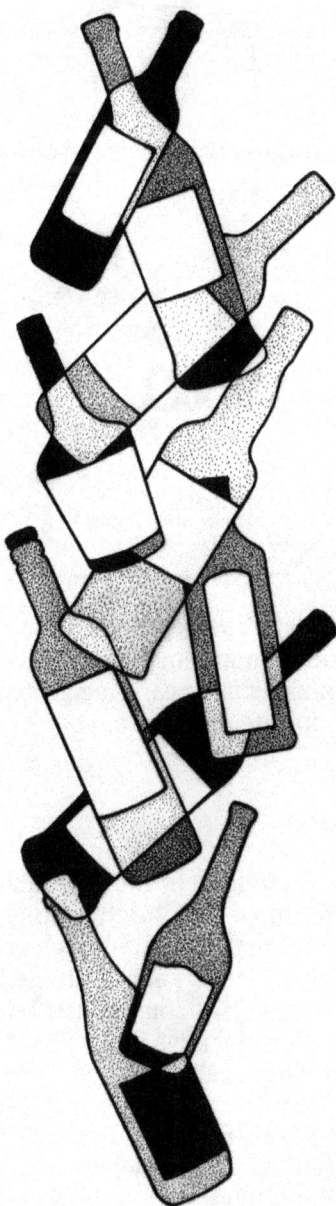

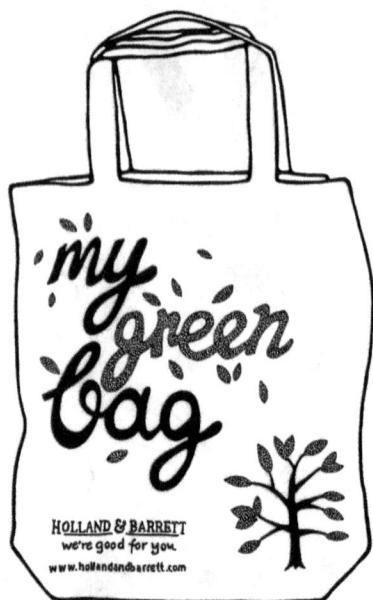

enthusiastic, if I danced around wearing avocado undies, playing percussion with the Avocado Pair. Maybe not. I would surely put them off their Mexxa nachos, enchilada or tostadas de chilli.

Ben enjoys the veggie quesadilla, jalapeño poppers, and the avocado and mozzarella salad. I commented that jalapeño poppers (breaded sliced green jalapeños stuffed with cream cheese and served with peach salsa) would be a *really good name* for a Mexican band. He gave me his vaguely-amused-musician-look, then gave me the oil of evening primrose and Ginkgo Biloba, which I had asked him to purchase from Holland & Barrett. The plastic jars were in a sweet little bleached cotton bag, with 'My Green Bag' printed on both sides in green. But I couldn't be too overjoyed, because I had visions of using it for carrying green bottles to a recycling skip in the car park opposite *our* house.

Sunday 3rd

Autumn yellow sunshine kissed me softly on both cheeks, as I plodded to the bird table with bread and peanuts, first thing this morning. The bright-bonny-blue-sky welcomed me to a fresh, new autumnal day. Squirrels were bouncing along tree branches, and busy burying their peanuts in the lawn. A magpie squawked, 'Good morning ma'am.' Well, that's what I like to he imagine he said. He was probably saying, 'I'll have that crust in a minute, hurry up and push-off indoors, so I can grab it before those pigeons get their greedy little beaks on it!'

I put the kettle on, and watched the magpie descend onto the bird table, for the crust he felt he had earned. After feeding the cats, feeding myself boiled egg and toast soldiers, then wading through last night's washing-up, I felt *so* worn out that I decided I had earned a treat. It was *after eight*, after all, so I awarded myself two little darkly deliciously divine squares of delightfully cold, crispy, minty heaven.

This afternoon I leafed through the Yellow Moon catalogue. I thought I may order the Woodland foam stickers; trees, acorns, owls, foxes, hedgehogs, squirrels..... Or the autumn leaf stickers; bright reds, yellows, greens or oranges. They will all look good on black card. I have a supply of A3 and A5 black card, ready for card making. A creative-card-making-witch *always* has black card. I should have mentioned this in my witchy book, but it is all finished now. *Done, done, done, completely completed.* If I keep having these thoughts I will just have to write another book; *More Love & Best Witches*, or *Lots of Love & Best Witches x x x.* Maybe a little book of recipes with illustrations. I used to enjoy baking delicious quiches, so I could write a cookery book entitled; *Loving Best Quiches.* Maybe not.

Anyway, for now I will think about Halloween, and making Happy Halloween cards for my witchy friends and little niece. I will order the Halloween foam stickers. The colours will look glowingly-effective on black card: purple and green spiders, purple bats, orange pumpkins, white ghosts and green witches. The black cats will be lost on a black background, so I'll stick them on the white envelopes, maybe add a green witch or spider.

I have some birthday cards to make too, so I'll order the foam, jigsaw puzzle shaped stickers, with a letter of the alphabet printed on the front of each piece. I can spell out HAPPY BIRTHDAY, or the birthday person's name, or both, or BEST WITCHES. And that reminds me, I must start my Disney

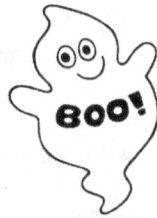

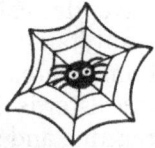

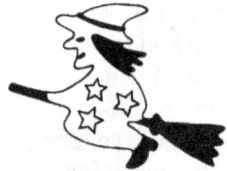

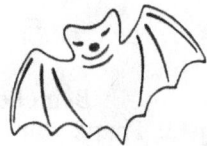

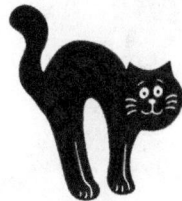

jigsaw puzzle soon. I can begin by piecing together my favourite Disney characters: The Aristocats, Alice in Wonderland, and so many more..... I don't know how I contain my excitement. The colourful jigsaw pieces would look good on black card; I could make greetings cards piecing together characters I think someone will like, when the whole puzzle is completed. The possibilities for creative fun are *simply endless* if you put your mind to it. If you have the energy to put your mind to anything.

It didn't take much energy to feel inspired by the Love Lavender catalogue, lavender everything: fragrant candles, cologne spray, talc, soap, pot pourri, Victorian sachets, body lotion, body wraps, home-ware..... I noticed many gifts I would *love* to order for family. My sister is going through the menopause, so she might appreciate a relaxing and soothing lavender gift. The lavender foot soak, with witch hazel and cooling peppermint, sounds an ideal gift for her too, because she has problems with her feet. The gardener collection looks good for auntie and uncle, who enjoy gardening. The collection has been especially created for gardeners, and formulated using Norfolk lavender and rosemary oils, with various blends of natural essential oils and herbs. The large lavender pillar candle would delicately fragrance a room, and set the mood for Ben's sister when she practises her yoga.

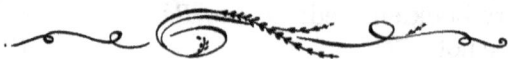

Ben checked my emails for me tonight. I received four; subject: Thank you for *Love & Best Witches*, from Ben's sister-in-law and three friends, all looking forward to reading the book. *Wonderful.*

I noticed in my newsletter from the Sussex and Kent M.E./CFS Society, that Russell Grant is a new patron. Great. I like Russell better than Cosmic Colin. I will ask Ben to email Colin Barton (the chairman of the society) if he will put an advert for my witchy book in their winter newsletter in time for Christmas. *Broomsticks crossed!!*

Monday 4th

9.30 a.m.   Just sitting.
Watching the squirrels in the sycamore trees.

9.34 a.m.   Just sitting.
Watching sycamore seeds flutter across the lawn.

9.35 a.m.   Just sitting.
Recalling the sycamore seed that fell into my peppermint tea, and floated, bobbing like a wooden rowing boat on dark seaweed-green waters.

9.42 a.m.   Just sitting.
Watching the second hand march around the face of the kitchen clock.

9.55 a.m.   Just sitting.
Wishing the plates and cutlery would wash themselves.

10.22 a.m.   Just sitting.
Watching Ben's shirts swirl round in the washing machine.

10.30 a.m.   Just sitting.
Watching the clouds float by, feeling lonely as a cloud, and poetic.....

JUST SITTING

Just sitting
Watching the clouds
Float by

Just sitting
Waiting for eggs
To fry

10.33 a.m.   I can't think of any more lines. Maybe something about waiting for pigs to fly... sigh...

10.34 a.m.   Try... Eye... Why... Die... Cry... Goodbye.

10.35 a.m.   I have words, but no lines.

10.36 a.m.   Just a couple of lines of an old song in my head, written in the 1940's by Cole Porter.

Every time we say goodbye, I die a little
Every time we say goodbye, I wonder why a little

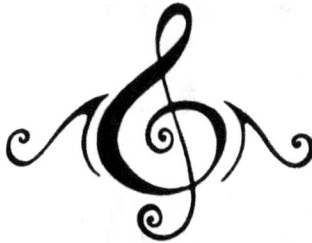

10.37 a.m.

Just sitting
With a song
In my head

I want to
Fall into
My comfortable
Bed

11.02 a.m

Just sitting
Listening to
A tick tock
Sound
As the hand
On the clock
Marches
Around

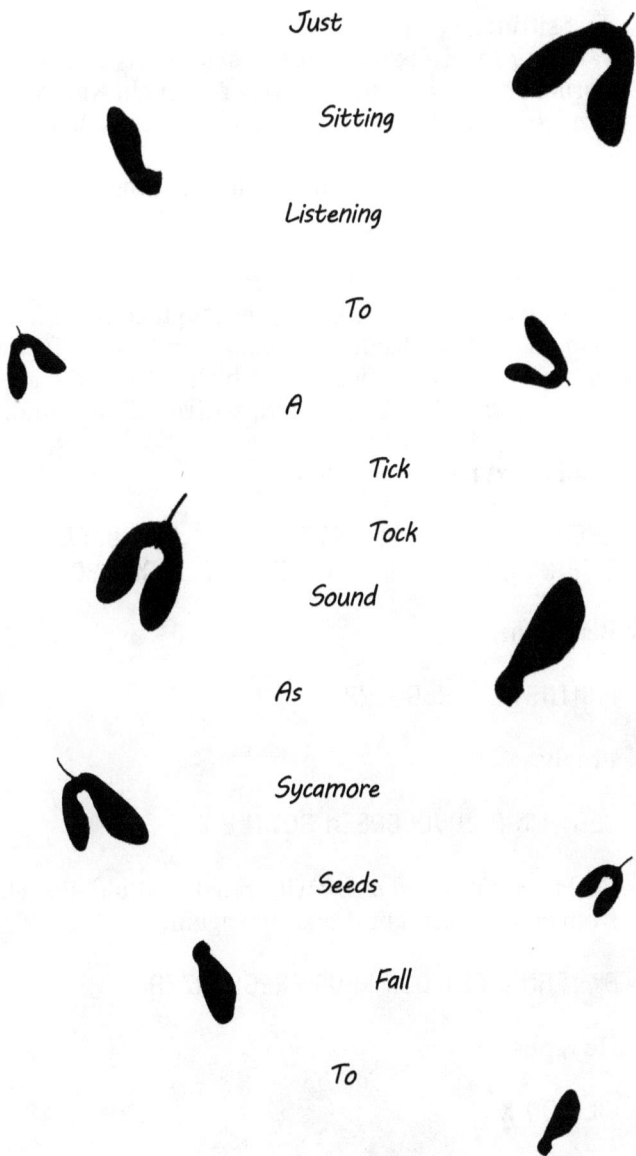

October

Just

Sitting

Listening

To

A

Tick

Tock

Sound

As

Sycamore

Seeds

Fall

To

The

Ground

11.15 a.m.   Just sitting.
             Wishing I were staring out to sea, in my house on the
             Cornish coast, next door to Dawn French, who may find
             a message in a bottle on her beach-front-garden.

11.16 a.m.   Trying not to think about bottle recycling skips on our
             front garden.

11.45 a.m.   *Hurrah! Hurrah! HURRAH!!!*
             A letter has arrived from our borough council: ..... blah
             blah..... waste collection team..... blah blah..... further to
             letters of objection received..... blah blah..... the site will
             not be installed..... blah..... alternative will be found.

11.46 a.m.   Send a text message to Ben:

             GREAT NEWS - GOT LETTER FROM B-COUNCIL TO SAY
             SITE WILL NOT BE INSTALLED - WELL DUN YOU X

11.47 a.m.   Ben replies:

             FANTASTIC - BUBBLY?

11.48 a.m.   I reply:

             YES - IN A LUVLI GREEN BOTTLE X

11.50 a.m.   Feel *very tired* and *weak* with relief. I would like a break
             from cooking tonight. I text Ben again:

             B - CAN U GET OUR FAVE FRESH PIZZA?

11.52 a.m.   He replies:

             WILL DO X

1.00 p.m.   Just sitting.
             Smiling.

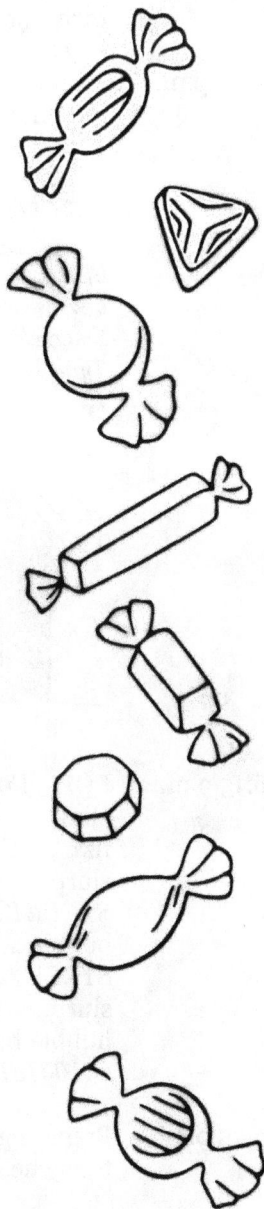

1.02 p.m.	I'm wearing my bottle-green hair scrunchie. The colour doesn't bother me any more, because I am *cool*. Cool as a fresh green cucumber. Cool as the olive green glassware in Weekly Wife. Cool as a Rovers Return bottle bank celebrating 50 years of *Coronation Street*, in my R.N.L.I. Catalogue.
1.20 p.m.	Reading TV mag. *Coronation Street* should be good tonight; Carla turns up at Pete's AA meeting, Tina confides in Rita, and Kevin bonds with Jack.
1.22 p.m.	You never see anyone eating chocolate on *Coronation Street*.
1.23 p.m.	If there were a soap called *Quality Street*, they would be eating chocolate all the time.
1.24 p.m.	Hmmm...
1.25 p.m.	It's a long time since I enjoyed some Quality Street.
1.26 p.m.	Hmmmmm.....
1.27 p.m.	Text Ben:

CAN YOU ADD SMALL BOX OF
QUALITY STREET TO SHOPPIN LIST
PLEASE?

1.35 p.m.	Ben replies:

OK

1.46 p.m. Reading my stars in Weekly Wife. Cosmic Colin says I thrive on peace. You are so right Col – lots of peace.

1.48 p.m. Inspired by Cosmic Colin, the squirrels, and the beach hut gifts in my R.N.L.I. catalogue.....

OCTOBER

Blessed peace and harmony
Leaves are falling from the tree
Squirrels hide their tiny nuts
Time to close up your beach huts

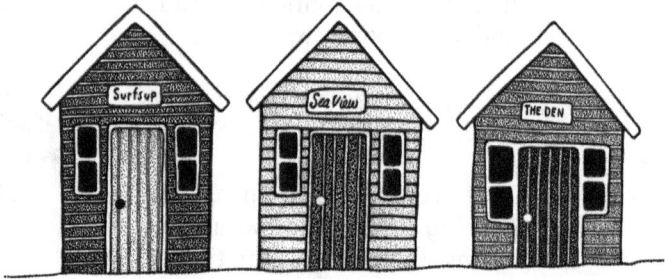

6.15 p.m. POP! Fizz fizz fizz..... bubble bubble..... sparkle..... clink..... *Cheers!*..... slurp slurp..... fizz..... sparkle..... fizz..... *CONGRATULATIONS!*..... bubble..... sparkle..... slurp..... slurp..... *HERE'S TO OUR QUIET LITTLE STREET*..... clink..... fizz fizz..... slurp..... bubble bubble..... *AND FIFTY YEARS OF CORONATION STREET*..... sparkle sparkle..... bubble..... fizz..... fizz..... slurp..... *HERE'S TO LOVE AND BEST WITCHES*..... hubble bubble..... clink..... fizz..... *AND ALL WHO SAIL ON THEIR BROOMSTICKS!*..... fizz..... fizz..... *CHEERS!*

6.35 p.m. Preparing salad to go with pizza. Fizzy bubbles have gone to my head, and I drop a tomato on the kitchen floor.

6.36 p.m.   Just sipping.
             Staring at tomato on green floor tiles, and bubbling with
             creativity.

TOMATO

There's a tomato
On the kitchen floor
Looking all forlorn
Like a small red ball
On a well mown lawn

6.39 p.m.   Just sipping.
             Staring at a Neapolitan-style pizza and sparkling with
             creativity.

PIZZA

Sweet Italian tomatoes
A rich rounded flavour
They burst with basil freshness
Ready just to savour

Pair ruby red tomatoes
With ricotta cheese
An indulgent blend, delicious
Only there to please

7.15 p.m.   Just sitting.
             Happily digesting.

7.17 p.m.   Sainsbury's didn't have any small boxes of Quality Street,
             so Ben had to get a large one – what a shame. I poured the
             sweets into a bowl so we could enjoy the shiny, colourful
             and tempting wrappers. Delicious golden shades: the toffee
             penny, toffee deluxe, caramel swirl. Gorgeous greens,
             strawberry reds and fuchcia pink, magical purple and blue.

7.18 p.m.	I chose my favourites; the purple one, the green triangle and a coconut éclair. Ben chose his favourites; the toffee finger, the green triangle and an orange chocolate crunch.
7.20 p.m.	As I unwrapped *the green triangle,* I wondered if there is a street called Quality Street. Ben was sitting at his computer, so I asked him if he would search on the internet for me. He discovered there are a few Quality Streets in Scotland and one in Surrey.
ME:	I think the people who live in Quality Street should paint their front doors the same colours as these chocolate wrappers.
BEN:	Maybe they do!
ME:	If I lived in Quality Street, instead of Orchard Street, I would always have these chocolates in my fruit bowl instead of apples. My front door would be the same colour as *the green triangle.* I would have strawberry red window frames and bright blue curtains; fuchcia pink window boxes full of deep-purple and yellow pansies, and a big squashy toffee coloured three piece *sweet.* What do you think?
BEN:	Yes, very nice dear (Basil Fawlty voice).
ME:	In our back garden we could have *quality* patio furniture, painted gold, with a large yellow umbrella. And colourful flowers in pots and hanging baskets. And roses everywhere. I don't know the names of many flowers, but know lots of names of roses, and their colours. Mum was always talking about her roses.
BEN:	That's wonderful dear (Basil Fawlty voice).
ME:	We could spend hours of *quality* time in our garden on a *Nice Day* (pink rose), counting our *Blessings* (pink rose) and celebrating *The Gift of Life* (orange rose).

On a day like today we could enjoy a *Champagne Moment* (pink rose). I do love to celebrate a *Special Occasion* (yellow rose) full of *Congratulations* (pink rose).

BEN: How lovely (Basil Fawlty voice).

ME: I could do my Disney jigsaw puzzle outside in the fresh air, maybe start with Alice in Wonderland in the rose garden – all my roses would inspire me. There's a red rose named Peter Pan!

BEN: *Fascinating* dear.
I expect you'll be wanting Cadbury's Roses chocolates when we've eaten all the Quality Street (Basil Fawlty voice).

ME: Of course Basil. I suggest you write that down before you forget, you know what you are like (Basil Fawlty's wife's voice).

BEN: Certainly *dear,* I'm making a note right now *dear.*

7.30 p.m. Just sitting.
Enjoying the drama, tension and sweetness in *Coronation Street.*

7.31 p.m. Just sitting.
Enjoying the delicious taste and sweetness of Quality Street.

8.05 p.m. There's a knock at our front door. A neighbour, Eileen, has called to say, 'Thanks and *well done* for your effort.'

8.07 p.m. Ben pours more champagne.

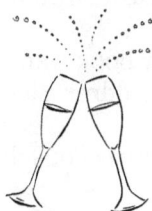

Tuesday 5th

Received a lovely reply from Colin Barton of the Sussex and Kent M.E./CFS Society today, saying he would happily include the advert for my witchy book in the winter edition of his newsletter. *Wonderful!*

I parcelled up a copy of *Love & Best Witches* with a letter of thanks, a cheque for thirty five pounds, and a donation to Colin's charity. I'm looking forward to seeing the advert for *my book*. Finally done. Completely completed.

Christmas gifts arrived too from animal charities; the P.D.S.A. and R.S.P.C.A., so it was quite an exciting day. The bed socks for my friends who have M.E., were lovely and soft. I will put a pair in my niece's Christmas stocking, she will like the little bear motif, because he's holding a big red heart. I enjoyed sniffing the scented gifts for relatives, and Ben's *HOT! HOT! HOT!* collection of chilli sauces were nostril tingling too.

When he returned from playing at the Mexxa Mexxa restaurant tonight, wearing his jazzy-blues shirt and tired musician's smile, he mentioned that he was going to do a gig with a couple of African percussion players next month. I had browsed through a clothes catalogue earlier; lots of jackets and jumpers in shades of cherry, peacock, fuchsia, rust and electric blue. They were also available in black.

ME: If you form a new band with the African players, you could call yourselves, Also Available In Black!

BEN: Yes dear. Very inspired *dear* (Basil Fawlty voice).

ME: Is Stephen the drummer still playing with Black Pizza, supported by Limp Salad?

BEN: Yes! *Hahaha* (Basil Fawlty laugh).

ME: The witch in my book wants to form a band called Black Sabbat or the Cauldron Sisters.

BEN: That's *simply marvellous* dear.

Wednesday 6ᵗʰ

I woke up quietly cackling to myself this morning, after a night of performing with the rock band, Black Sabbath. I was playing cauldron shaped drums, wearing a big black pointy hat, and black rock star clothes. My drum sticks were magical wands made from willow, and starry sparks flew around when I hit the toms. After the concert, I had a late dinner with the band at Black Pizza Hut, where they served up black pizzas with limp salad.

My day was far less active than my night, I felt tired and floppy. Well, more tired and floppy than usual; and I became so engrossed in a daydream about playing with a rock band, that I let my toast burn, and had to put another slice under the grill. My hands were weak and achy, after yesterday's parcelling-up and opening-of-parcels, so I almost had black toast with limp hands for breakfast.

Luckily I didn't have to prepare veg for dinner because Ben sent me a text message:

9.05 a.m. GOIN OUT 4 INDIAN AFTER WORK X

9.06 a.m. OH GOOD – HAVE A DELISH MEAL – C U LATER X

10.20 a.m. Text from Jayne:

HEY WITCHY FRIEND – HOW R U ? I-M EXHAUSTED BUT GOOD – MY FRIEND DAVE IS A LITTLE BETTER BUT HAS A LONG WAY TO GO – BLESS HIM – SLEEPY HUGS XXX

10.22 a.m. I reply:

HI SLEEPY WITCH – I-M A WORN OUT WITCH TODAY – WAITING TO HEAR IF AFME WILL REVIEW MY BOOK – GOT AN AD IN KENT AND SUSSEX ME NEWSLETTER – HURRAH – SEND MY BEST WITCHES TO DAVE – AND HEALING HUG 4 U XXX

Thursday 7ᵗʰ

Autumn's must-have Mavala nail polish shade has arrived; the milk-chocolaty shade is chic on the shortest nails and gorgeous on toes – says Wendy of Weekly Wife. Max Factor's Coco Crazy Trio eye-shadow is shades of milk, plain and white chocolate. Delicious *must-haves.*

Lush do a double-choc lip tint with ingredients including; cocoa butter, black treacle, brandy, dark chocolate and brazil nut oil. And a lip balm; Whipstick, made with shea butter, honey, tangerine oil and dark chocolate. Surely you would be licking them off your lips!

Lush also make toffee and chocolate bubble bars, for bath-time fun; a mint chocolate sugar scrub, and a chocolate and vanilla lip scrub. I must start my *must-have* list for Santa, he likes to shop at Lush for me.

2.00 p.m.   Start *must-have* list.

2.04 p.m.   Must have chocolate.

2.05 p.m.   Ben ate the last of the Quality Street last night.

2.06 p.m.   Text Ben:

HELP – MUST HAVE CHOC – WE NEED SOYA MILK TOO X

2.10 p.m.   CERTAINLY DEAR – ROSES CHOC?

2.11 p.m.   YES – THANX BASIL X

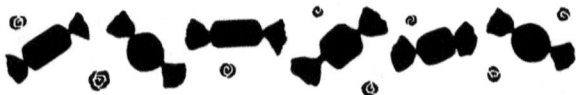

2.14 p.m.   Browsing through P.D.S.A. Christmas gift catalogue, to take my mind off chocolate.

2.16 p.m.   Ooh! I like their roomy canvas shoppers. The colours and design will perfectly match the fleecy blankets on the cat beds. Chocolate brown with cream paw prints, and cream with chocolate brown paw prints.

2.17 p.m.	No. *No, no, no.* I will not think about the colour of milk chocolate. I will think about paw prints.
2.18 p.m.	The canvas shoppers will match the paw prints I painted on one of Ben's guitars. They are the colours of three of our departed cats. Ginger, black and grey.
2.46 p.m.	And the shoppers will match the paw prints I drew on a white tee-shirt, with orange, black and grey fabric pens.
3.10 p.m.	And the black paw prints embroidered on a red hand towel.
4.17 p.m.	And the muddy paw prints on our green kitchen tiles.
4.18 p.m.	I am visualising the colours: orange, black, grey, red and green.
4.20 p.m.	And the colour yellow. The yellow paw print design on a purple background, on the cat food tin.
5.00 p.m.	I painted paw prints on my arm with henna once. The henna looked like chocolate in a tube. *No, no, no.* I'm thinking: yellow, purple, black, grey, orange, green and red.
5.10 p.m.	I'm hanging my brown owl jumper in the wardrobe, next to a black velvet dress. But I'm not thinking brown. I'm thinking black. Black as the night. Black as a witch wearing her black pointy hat and velvet cloak. Black as her cat. Black as Black Forest gateaux.... *No, no, no.* I'm thinking green. Forests of green. Lovely green trees. Green and black. Green and Black chocolate bars. All sorts of delicious flavours: mint, butterscotch, strawberry, orange..... *No, no, no.* I will think of orange. Mountains of big fat oranges. Lots of juicy segments. Chocolate orange, with lots of crispy segments, cold from the fridge. So chocolaty. So orangy..... *No, no, no.* I will think of the orange pepper in the fridge. Firm and fresh. There's a red one too. Red, red, red. Red as a tomato. Red as a strawberry. Red as the filling of Lindt strawberry cheesecake chocolate

bar..... *No, no, no*. There's a yellow pepper in the fridge with the red and orange pepper. I'm thinking yellow. Yellow as lemons hanging from a lemon tree in sunny Spain. Yellow as daffodils in the springtime. Yellow as the double yellow lines in the road. Double yellow. Double chocolate gateaux..... *No, no, no*. I'm thinking yellow, yellow as the paw prints in a purple background on the tin of cat food. Purple. I like purple. The colour of psychic ability. Witches love to wear purple. The purple of Cadbury's chocolate wrappers. Witches love Cadbury's or Green and Black chocolate bars............................ I give up.

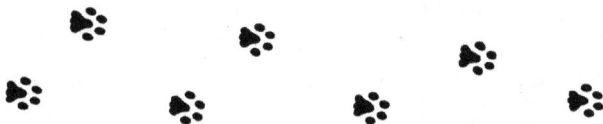

6.10 p.m.   Ben arrives home. He is my knight with a shiny carrier bag, full of chocolates and soya milk.

6.12 p.m.   Mmm..... Hazel in caramel..... Country fudge..... Strawberry dream.

6.13 p.m.   Shiny colourful wrappers – like Quality Street. I think I will collect them to make shiny colourful Christmas cards; they will look good on black card, with the Christmas stickers I ordered from Yellow Moon catalogue last year. And a creative-card-making-witch *always* has lots of black card.

Friday 8th

      I perched my creaky old bones on my creaky old wooden garden bench; a small pile of today's Christmas gift catalogues sat beside me. The afternoon autumn sunshine was quite hot, and for a while it felt like summertime. I sipped my steaming peppermint tea and smiled, as though I were savouring the last of the summer wine. A soft breeze blew the pages of ACE catalogue over for me, which was quite handy because I still felt very tired and floppy today. As I studied Christmas card scenes: waving Santas and penguins, reindeer flying, and happy Christmas shoppers shopping; a robin bobbed on the fence nearby.

ME: Hi Bobby, you're chirpy today.

BOBBY: *What are you like,* I'm always chirpy! (robin language).

A ladybird landed on a picture of an easy-to-assemble, super-thick and bushy, smoky mountain pine tree, complete with *real* pine cones. I noticed she had lots of spots on her shiny red wings, instead of three or four.

ME: Hi Dotty, you look pretty, is that the latest ladybird fashion?

DOTTY: *What are you like,* of course it is! (ladybird language).

A squirrel nibbled on a peanut at the nearby bird table, as I studied the choice of festive garlands: holly and berry, cream and gold, or black and silver.

ME: Hi Nutty, I hope you remember where you've hidden your nuts.

NUTTY: *What are you like,* us squirrels always remember! (squirrel language).

My next door neighbour was hanging out his washing and probably thinking - *What is she like!*
I know what *I* like. A Christmas card that makes me cackle; Santa's washing hanging on a washing line.

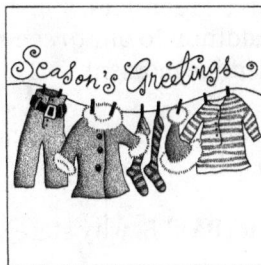

Saturday 9th

Bloom catalogue arrived today, full of beautifully colourful silk flower arrangements and small silk trees in pots. I've never liked plastic or silk flowers, but since I've had M.E., the thought of plants that don't need tending have a certain appeal. A certainly huge appeal. A *blooming* good idea!

The ruby and white winter arrangements were *most* appealing; pure white roses and gardenias in full bloom, displayed against a background of mixed winter foliage and red berries. The festive red berry garlands and deep red amaryllis were lovely. The witchy, black phalaenopsis orchid caught my eye, described in the catalogue as exotic and spell binding. The witch in my book would have adored one of those. She would have liked the magical Maidenhair fern *and* the Asplenium fern too.

The silk trees in pots were attractive, especially the olive tree. The catalogue suggested I think of dazzling white cottages over-looking the blue Aegean, and brightly painted fishing boats bobbing in the harbour..... *it's a long way from an English winter, but our new olive tree will make your Mediterranean dream a little more real. Beautifully detailed for complete realism ~ from the silvery leaves to the gnarled trunk ~ it's ideal for the kitchen, conservatory or hall, in fact anywhere you fancy a Shirley Valentine moment.*

There's no room in our tiny kitchen, for a Mediterranean olive tree in a pot; just room in a cupboard, for a jar of Moroccan black olives and Manzanilla green olives. We haven't got a hall or a conservatory, but there may be room in the corner of the bathroom. The tree would feel at home with my overgrown ivy and spider plants, avocado green bathroom suite, bracken-green towels, seaweed and mint Lush soaps, olive conditioning shampoo, lime green toothbrush holder to match the smiley green frogs and seahorses, and Botanics aromatherapy oils in olive green jars. I'm sure Ben will be *simply enamoured* with a new addition to our *green peaceful* bathroom. And I often fancy a Shirley Valentine moment.

ME: I'd like an olive tree in the bathroom, so I can have Shirley Valentine moments.

BEN: No comment (Basil Fawlty stare).

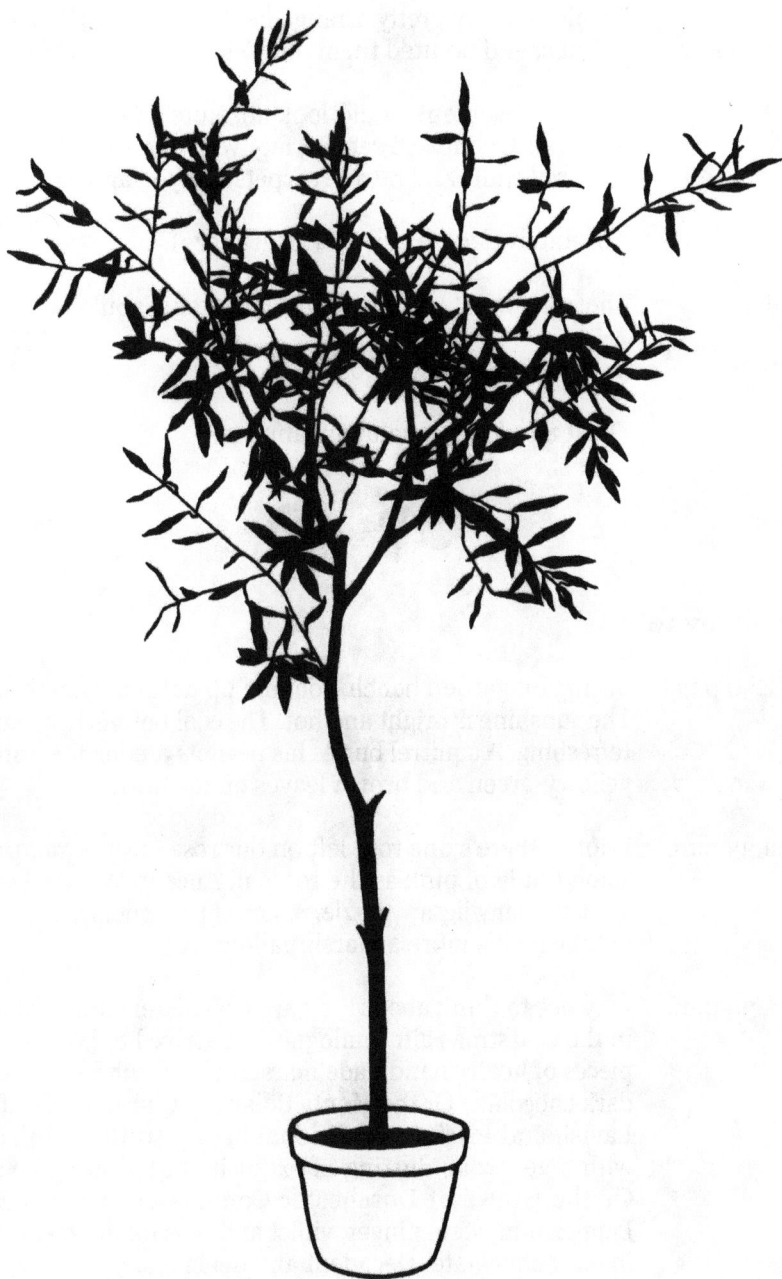

I noticed a very pretty arrangement of silk roses, in shades of yellow and orange, and pointed them out to Ben.

ME: This arrangement would look absolutely fabulous in our house in Quality Street. Perfect with the squashy toffee sofa, red walls and purple carpets. Do you agree?

BEN: Absolutely *dear* (Basil Fawlty grimace).

ME: There's a yellow rose named Absolutely Fabulous.

BEN: Is there a Verity Red rose?

ME: That *would* be absolutely fabulous!

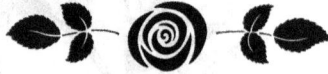

Sunday 10th

12.30 p.m.   Sitting on garden bench, soaking up autumn sun-beams. The sunshine is bright and hot. The cool breeze, beautifully refreshing. A squirrel buries his peanuts among the crinkly yellowy-green and brown leaves on the lawn.

12.33 p.m.   I notice there's one rose left on our rose bush, *exactly* the same shade of pink as the roses in Alice in Wonderland's garden, in my jigsaw puzzle. A sort of pale bubblegum pink. Or maybe it's more a marshmallow pink.

12.34 p.m.   I try not to think about the dark chocolate marshmallows in the Christmas gift catalogue that arrived today. Twenty pieces of luxury handmade marshmallow, enrobed in thick dark chocolate. Or the Monty Bojangles Chocolaty Truffles. Lavish and luscious traditional luxury truffles, finished with a generous dusting of exquisite bitter-sweet cocoa. Or the House of Dorchester Connoisseur Chocolates. Peppermint, stem ginger, violet and rose fondant, covered in dark chocolate. Decadent and delicious.

12.35 p.m. I will write some verse, inspired by my rose. I fancy some rose fondant. *No,no,no.*

12.36 p.m. I recall a squirrel I once saw, pick one of our pink roses, pull the petals off one by one, and eat them. He looked like he was enjoying the taste. I wonder............. *no, no, no.* I will not be tempted to eat my last rose. Maybe just one petal.......... *no, no, no.* What if someone saw me. What *would* the neighbours think! I will write verse. I will think about delicate pink petals falling like like tear drops.......... that sort of thing.

12.50 p.m. OCTOBER ROSE

October rose
You remind me
Of July
Soon
Your petals
Will
Fall
Where autumn
Leaves
Lie

Delicate
Pink tear drops
Flutter
Down
To rest
On
Mother Nature's
Old
Brown
Cheek

1.12 p.m. Reading in Weekly Wife about our bodies using sunlight to help our skin produce vitamin D; it's found in very few foods so it's important to get some sunlight. Wendy suggests you get twenty to thirty minutes of sun, two or three times a week, during the months April to September. I will remember this *next* year. I can forget about it now, but a few October rays are doing me good. I will enjoy them before it's too chilly to sit outside.

2.10 p.m.   Receive text message from Jayne. Her little sister loves Halloween, so I recently sent her a copy of my witchy book:

HEY KIND WITCH, I-VE BEEN POOPD BUT JUST WANTED 2 LET U KNOW THAT MANDY WAS THRILLED THAT U SENT HER UR BOOK – SHE HAS ALREADY STARTED READING IT – WITCHY HUGS X X X

2.11 p.m.   I reply:

HI POOPD WITCH – THAT-S GREAT – HOPE MANDY ENJOYS THE BOOK – HAPPY WITCH HUGS X X X

Unbeknown to me, Ben asked his sister if she would review my book on the Amazon books website. Julia had replied, saying she would love to, so I texted to thank her this morning. This afternoon I received a reply:

2.30 p.m.   HI VERITY, THANKS FOR MESSAGE – I-M LOOKING FORWARD TO WRITING REVIEW – WILL DO IT NEXT WEEK – PAUL IS GOING TO MIRANDA-S TODAY AND WILL GIVE BOOK TO KIRA – MAYBE SHE COULD DO A REVIEW TOO – LOTS OF LOVE, JULIA X X X

2.31 p.m.   Brilliant!

Monday 11th

A catalogue arrived from La Redoute. It was the JOYEUX NOEL Christmas edition 2010. The model on the cover looked very festive and jolly, wearing a sparkly sequin jacket and *isn't-Christmas-a-fabulous-time* smile. I removed the plastic cover, and as I browsed through the fabulously-festive-fashions, I felt some verse coming on.....

Things in shiny packets
Girls in sequin jackets

..... then I lost interest. I was much more inspired by a surprise package from my friend Jim, who like me, has had M.E. for many years. He writes wonderful humorous verse, so I put two of his poems in my witchy book, and thought I would surprise him with a copy as soon as it was printed.

I was *most delighted* with his beautiful art nouveau card, thanking me for the book, and saying he enjoyed it so much he couldn't put it down. Lovely! He also sent a poem, inspired by his baby grand-daughter Isabelle Grace, with a photo of her dressed in a baby Halloween costume; tiny black dress with a hood, stripy red and white tights, and black booties. I can't recall when I last cackled so much, and I'm going to have it professionally framed.

A DAY IN THE LIFE OF A VERY YOUNG CHILD

A little girl called Issy
Is kept very, very busy
Learning all the things a baby has to do
How to call on dad and mum
When she has an empty tum
Or get some comfort when she's feeling blue

And if that's not enough
There is lots of other stuff
That mum's decided Issy ought to do
For mum has had a whim
That Issy should learn to swim
And learn to enjoy poetry too

So every single day
Is filled with lots of play
And learning to get everything just right
But all things Issy enjoys
Are just mum's cunning ploys
To make sure Issy sleeps right through the night

I was *most inspired* by a short story Jim had written for me, entitled; The Hunt for the Unicorn, with photos too. The unicorn hunt was part of a gala, organised by his wife Pauline in the summer. The trail to find the unicorn was set in nearby woods, and looked *fabulous fairytale fun* for all the family.

I enjoyed the photos of adults and children, dressed as a troll, water-sprite, pixies, fairies, a wizard putting on a magic show. There was a little white pony wearing a unicorn horn too. As I gazed at the miniature wood at the end of our garden, fairy sparkles of inspiration twinkled like little stars in my eyes, and I wrote some verse in my head. Mary purred by my side, my *furry-tail* princess.

THE HUNT FOR THE UNICORN

We're hunting for the unicorn
In the woods, so deep
Tread carefully and whisper
When the fairies are asleep

Beware of the hairy troll
Who wears huge scary boots
Wave your wand and run away
Avoiding big tree roots

Beware too, of the water sprite
With water, she will spray
Just give her a big onion
And she'll guide you on your way

The pixies and the dryads
Will tell you where to go
Then you'll meet a wizard
Who'll put on a magic show

You may be feeling tired by now
Excited, but you yawn
Then before you know it
You will find the unicorn

I have two text messages, sent by Ben, that I keep in my mobile phone, because they make me smile every time I go through my messages for a deleting session:

ALWAYS BE YOURSELF – UNLESS YOU CAN BE A UNICORN – THEN ALWAYS BE A UNICORN – ANON

A BOOK FELL ON MY HEAD – I ONLY HAVE MY SHELF TO BLAME

Tuesday 12th

HURRAH! Received *another* surprise parcel from my friend Len, who also has a lovely baby granddaughter, Eleanor. He writes charming poetry, and I put one in my witchy book.

When I opened my parcel I found a delightful card (a photo of a ginger cat) congratulating me on my book. In my book I had mentioned Len was a wizard friend, and in his card he said he had almost become one once; he wrote a poem at the time. There was a copy of the poem enclosed with the card, it made me quietly cackle.

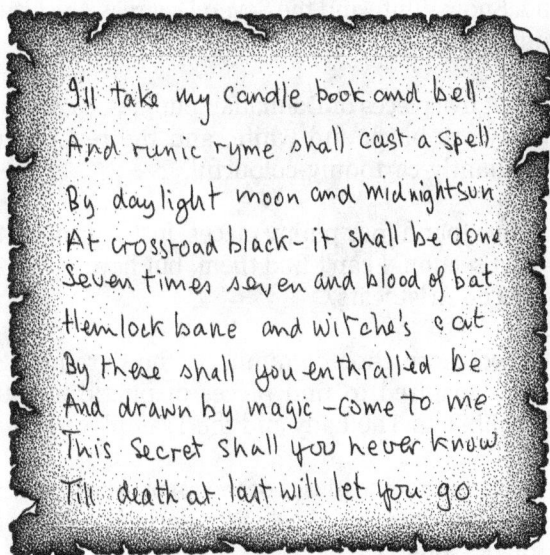

I'll take my candle book and bell
And runic ryme shall cast a spell
By daylight moon and midnightsun
At crossroad black – it shall be done
Seven times seven and blood of bat
Hemlock bane and witche's cat
By these shall you enthralled be
And drawn by magic – come to me
This secret shall you never know
Till death at last will let you go

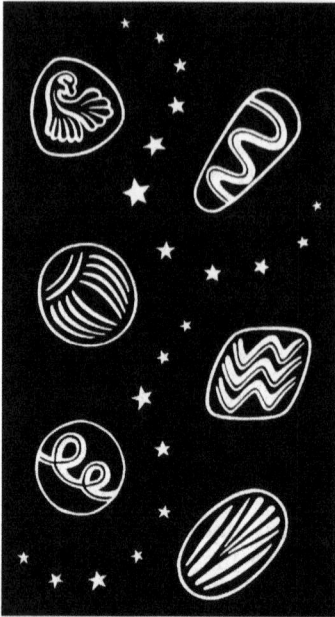

With the card and poem was a box of magic. A *beautiful* box of Black Magic. My witchy mouth watered as I removed the cellophane, lifted the lid, and enjoyed the aroma of dreamy dark chocolate caressing my senses. A delicious selection awaited my indulgence. I wondered which one I fancied first, they all looked *so tempting*.

As I popped the dreamy fudge into my mouth, I decided to enjoy a deliciously decadent afternoon; dark chocolate and a Disney jigsaw puzzle. What more could a girl want, apart from shoes. After removing the cellophane wrapper, I lifted the lid of the puzzle box, and hundreds of little colourful shapes awaited my pleasure. I noticed the face of one of the Aristocats, and decided to piece together my favourite characters first: The Aristocats, Dalmatian puppies, Lady and the Tramp, Alice in Wonderland, Snow White and the Seven Dwarves, the Little Mermaid, Peter Pan, and Bambi.

12.43 p.m.   Spot five pieces of Dalmatian puppies, easy to spot because they are black and white, and the rest of the puzzle is radiantly-cartoonly-colourful.

12.50 p.m.   Have found four puppy pieces, just four more to complete that section. I can't find them, but have found three pieces of The Aristocats.

1.02 p.m.   Need more choc..... mmm..... the Caramel Caress. I am now inspired to find pieces of puzzle in toffee shades; Bambi and The Lady and the Tramp's puppies.

1.27 p.m.   Have found five pieces of the raspberry-pink stripy cat and the pink roses in Alice's Wonderland garden, inspired by the Raspberry Parfait.

1.34 p.m.   Piecing together Peter Pan's orange hair and the orange
             Aristocat's bum, as the Orange sensation melts on my
             tongue.

2.00 p.m.   Have found some faces: Snow White, the Little Mermaid,
             Alice in Wonderland, Peter Pan, and one of the Dalmatian
             puppies; just a corner of puppy ear and a paw to find.
             I've *actually enjoyed* myself, even though my neck feels
             as stiff as a piece of good quality Ravensburger jigsaw
             puzzle. This could be my *new hobby*. Maybe I'll start
             collecting puzzles, I've seen some beautiful ones in
             Christmas gift catalogues: Winter Wonderland, Forest
             sanctuaries, Fairy dreams and celestial paintings. I could
             write a book entitled; *The Joy of Jigsaws*, and do little
             drawings of the most exciting parts to piece together. The
             possibilities for creative fun are *simply endless* if you put
             your mind to it. If you have the energy to put your mind
             to anything.

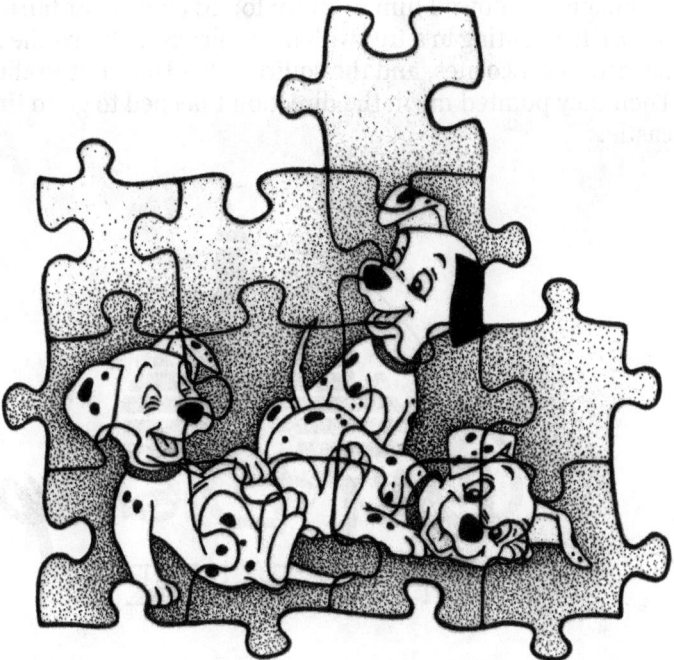

Wednesday 13th

LUCKY ME! *Another parcel* arrived today – Christmas gifts from the Love Lavender catalogue. The lavender scented candles smelt wonderfully fragrant, and I enjoyed a good old sniff of the Norfolk gardener collection (Auntie Jeanette and Uncle Keith will *love* it!). The muscle-rub, with eucalyptus, black pepper, and wintergreen oils, smelt healingly-good. The protecting weather cream, with shea butter, rosemary and lavender was a refreshing scent, and felt soothing on my finger tips. The hand scrub, with clary sage, lavender and aloe vera, had a foil cover over the top of the tube. I didn't want to remove it, in case it leaked when I sent it in the post, my hands aren't strong enough to screw tops back on tightly.

My neck and shoulders were very achy after yesterday's exciting afternoon, so I couldn't resist rubbing a little of the muscle-rub into my skin. I started to feel very sleepy. Then I closed my eyes......

I found myself wandering deep in a wood, searching for a raspberry-pink fairytale castle (with lots of turrets and flags, like at the beginning of Disney films). Peter Pan appeared, flying around my head, and I followed him until we found a group of fairies with bright orange hair, sitting in a tree with the squirrels. I offered the fairies Orange Sensation chocolates, and the squirrels the Hazelnut Praline chocolates. Then they pointed me in the direction I needed to go to find the Disney castle.

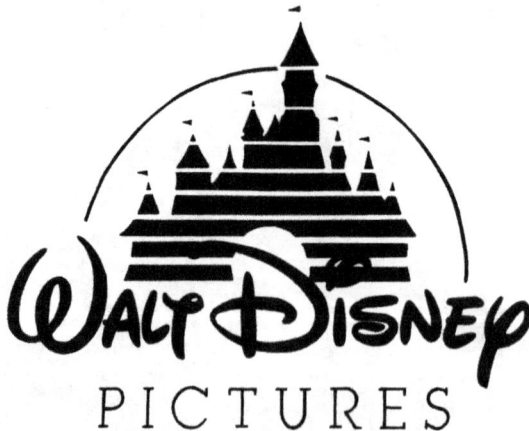

I continued my journey until I came to a crossroad, where I stopped, and scratched my head. I felt confused, I didn't know which path to take. Then I heard a rustling noise, and a dryad appeared from behind a tree, dressed in a leaf-green robe, with ivy in her hair. She didn't speak, just pointed to a yellow brick road.

I followed the yellow brick road, and after a while I met a wizard, wearing a purple pointy hat, and purple robe covered in silver moons and stars. I offered him Black Magic chocolates, and he chose the Raspberry Parfait. Suddenly, in the bright blue sky, a raspberry-pink stripy Cheshire cat appeared, under a rainbow. Then, with a flash from the wizard's wand, the cat turned into the Disney castle.

The wizard said I would find the Disney castle somewhere over the rainbow. I noticed the rainbow was the same colours as my Dorothy rainbow bath bomb, from Lush; yellow, orange and pink. Tiny fairies with translucent, rainbow wings, sat in the trees, singing; 'Somewhere over the rainbow'.

As I continued to stroll along the road, some of the yellow bricks became pink or orange, the moment I stepped on them. My rainbow road was leading me to the castle of my dreams. When I came to the end of the road, there was a man playing a white grand piano. He was dressed in blue sparkly seventies clothes, and wearing huge green sparkly spectacles. He smiled, like the Cheshire cat, and sang to me.

> *So goodbye yellow brick road*
> *Where the dogs of society howl*
> *You can't plant me in your penthouse*
> *I'm going back to my plough*
>
> *Back to the howling old owl in the woods*
> *Hunting the horny back toad*
> *Oh, I've finally decided my future lies*
> *Beyond the yellow brick road*

I sang along, and when the song ended, he asked if I had any requests. I asked for *Candle in the Wind.*

I finally found myself standing on the edge of a wonderful valley; Love Lavender valley, full of fields of lavender and swirling mists, scented with lavender. I stood breathing in the restful fragrance, watching the mists melt away; and there, in the middle of the valley appeared the raspberry-pink Disney castle, with purple turrets and little flags flying in a gentle breeze.

The scented mist made me feel so peaceful, I floated through the air, all the way down the valley to the castle entrance. The huge wooden doors opened, to reveal Alice in Wonderland's rose garden. Cadbury's Roses chocolates grew on rose bushes. I picked a Strawberry Dream, and wandered dreamily through the garden admiring red, yellow, orange, green, blue and purple roses, the same shades as Cadbury's Roses chocolate wrappers. Then I found myself in a clearing where a delightful scene met my eyes. A tea party. Alice sat at the end of a long wooden table, and her guests either side were: Peter Pan, Cinderella, the Little Mermaid, the Mad Hatter, Snow White and the Seven Dwarves. They were happily celebrating a very merry un-birthday, and invited me to join them, because it's unlucky to have thirteen guests at your tea party.

I sat down next to the Mad Hatter, who grinned at me and offered me a cup of tea. I smiled and accepted his offer, but as I sipped my tea, the whole scene became very still, like a photograph. Then the photograph became a jigsaw puzzle, and slowly started to fall apart. I woke up feeling fragile and a little puzzled, with a craving for chocolates, the urge to piece together the Alice in Wonderland part of my Disney jigsaw puzzle, *and* the need to listen to my Elton John CD's.

After dinner, despite my weary achy body, I put on an Elton John CD and sat down to complete more of my puzzle. I couldn't find any pieces of Alice, the Mad Hatter, or the White Rabbit. But I did find the Cheshire Cat's smiling face and more of his stripy tail.

I would have overdone it, and made myself painfully fatigued, but Cleopatra came to my rescue. She decided to climb into the puzzle box, trample on the puzzle pieces with her big white paws, then curl up for a long sleep. The box is similar in size and depth, to a cat litter tray; so I was *most relieved* that she didn't decide the puzzle pieces were multi-coloured cat litter, and *relieve* herself. As I watched her tummy rise and fall, her body like a large hairy cake in a cake tin (with self-raising fur) I wondered if she were having colourful Disney dreams; chasing Mickey Mouse, Donald Duck, or a white rabbit (wearing a waistcoat, with a large pocket watch, and late for a *very* important date) down a rabbit hole. Or maybe she was sitting in a tree, enjoying a conversation with a Cheshire cat, who says he'll take her to Alice's tea party.

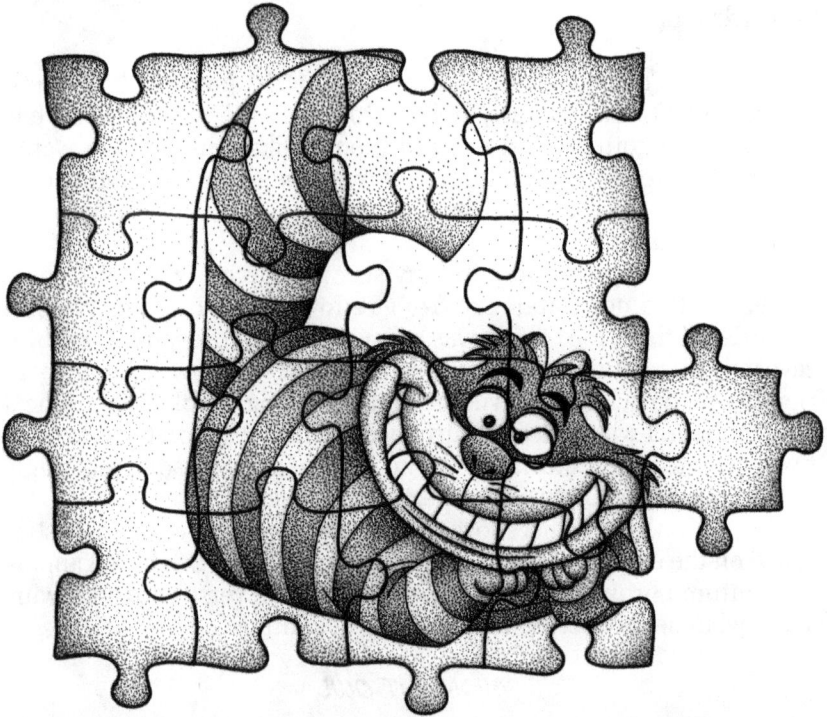

8.00 p.m.   Luxuriating in a deep lovingly warm bath, full of heavenly
             clouds of sparkling rainbow bubbles, pop, pop popping,
             with the scent of lavender and jasmine. Wild rose and
             raspberry tea-lights flicker in a tiny breeze from the
             bathroom window. I softly sing the chorus of a pop song
             by Elton John......

And it seems to me you lived your life
Like a candle in the wind
Never knowing who to cling to
When the rain set in
And I would have liked to have known you
But I was just a kid
Your candle burned out long before
Your legend ever did

Thursday 14th

Today was full of surprises. My botanical notelets, illustrated by Elizabeth Kerr, arrived from the M.E. Association. I had *completely* forgotten I had ordered them. I liked the delicate water-colours of flowers, they will be ideal for sending to auntie and garden loving friends. Good quality card too; a ripply texture, like *After Eight* minty chocolates.

I enjoyed opening my second parcel; woodland foam stickers, with a new catalogue from Yellow Moon. I had forgotten I had ordered them too. There was a fun selection: foxes, trees, rabbits, leaves, acorns, squirrels, pine cones, hedgehogs and owls. All my pen-friends who have M.E. are wildlife and pet loving people. When I next write to them, I will stick a colourful woodland sticker on the envelope. It will brighten their morning, to find a hedgehog or a squirrel, hiding under a pile of rectangular white and manilla leaves.

My little niece loves owls, so when I next write I will stick an owl on the envelope. Maybe a lime green tree with bright red apples, or an autumn brown leaf too. Louise wrote some verse with a drawing of an owl in her last letter, both were *so* delightful.

MIDNIGHT OWL

Eyes shining like lanterns
in the night sky,
Feathers ruffling in the midnight
breeze,
Wings beating to the rhythm of
the night.

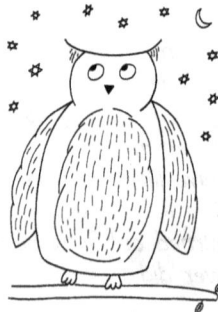

The free mystery gift from the P.D.S.A. was delightful too. A large, soft and velvety Christmas stocking; deep reds, blues and greens, with a cat design. The gifts I had ordered from the charity were delayed. I thought hard, but I couldn't recall what they were, maybe I had ordered just one gift, or some cards. My memory is like a *very leaky* cauldron as the festive season approaches.

I decided the Christmas stocking would be perfect for my niece, who loves her cats. Mystery gifts are often a *huge* disappointment: foul smelling soaps in a fancy cardboard box, a horrible plastic mac, miniature cheese grater, set of murderous looking knives, make-up purse with a *revolting* design, cheap looking *ugly* pendant, black plastic bottle stopper.....

My best surprise of the day, was Ben's sister's beautiful review of my book, on the Amazon books website. Ben printed it out for me when he came home from work, and I was *thrilled*. I reached for my mobile phone as soon as I read it.

6.15 p.m.   OOH, THANX JULIA FOR YOUR WONDERFUL REVIEW – I SO APPRECIATE THE TIME, THOUGHT, AND EFFORT YOU PUT INTO IT – BIG WITCHY HUG XXX

6.20 p.m.   Julia replied:

THANKS – IT WAS A PLEASURE TO WRITE IT AND I HOPE IT SELLS LOTS OF COPIES SO PLENTY OF PEOPLE GET THE FUN OF READING IT – KIRA IS IN THE MIDDLE OF READING IT AND LOVES IT TOO – BEST WITCHES, LOVE AND HUGS – JULIA XXX

8.00 p.m.   Sitting in bath smiling. So happy with my *first* review.

8.05 p.m.   Still smiling. Really pleased Julia's little granddaughter Kira is enjoying my book, it would be great if she could write a review from a child's point of view.

8.20 p.m.   Still in bath, singing.

So goodbye yellow brick road
Where the dogs of society howl
La la la la penthouse

La la la la la plough

8.25 p.m.　　*Goodbye Norma Jean*
Though I never knew you at all
La la la la la
La la la la la la

11.30 p.m.　　In bed dreaming. Julia, Kira, Louise and I are dressed as witches. But we're not wearing raven black; our clothes, pointy hats and pointy boots are shades of lavender, and Louise has her pet midnight owl perched on her shoulder. In the woods, we meet Marilyn Monroe, and Elton John, who has the Cheshire cat sitting on his shoulder. We offer them some of our Raspberry Parfait chocolates, then we all skip happily along the yellow brick road, singing about visiting a wizard.

Friday 15th

After breakfast I got stuck into some decorating. Well, not *exactly decorating*. Not papering, or repainting peeling walls. More like peeling the backing off some of my woodland stickers, and sticking them on the fridge door. It was a lot more enjoyable, and a lot less effort than decorating. I knew the wildlife in my garden would approve, if they popped in through the cat flap for a viewing.

9.15 a.m.　　I watched a squirrel, perched on the corner of our bird table, feeding on a peanut. Her little grey cheeks munching *madly*, fluffy tail quivering.

9.17 a.m.　　Inspired, I stuck a smiley squirrel on the fridge door. While I admired my effort, I recalled hearing foxes last night, with their strange spooky, breathy bark. So of course I felt inspired to peel the backing off a fox next.

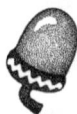

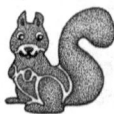

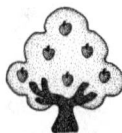

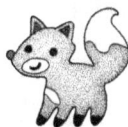

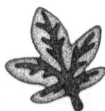

9.18 a.m.	Feeling a little sticker-happy, I added an acorn, leaf , and an apple tree.
9.20 a.m.	I admired my work again. A job *well done.*
9.21 a.m.	I smiled at the amusing quotes on the fridge magnets - Christmas gifts from thoughtful friends.

**Cats are like chocolates,
it's hard to have just one.**

**Friends are like fancy
chocolates, it's what's
inside that's special.**

9.22 a.m.	A strong gust of October wind blew the cat flap wide open. Purrdita flew into the kitchen with a greeny-yellow leaf stuck to her tabby coat.
9.23 a.m.	I shivered and thought it was time for another warming mug of something tasty. The squirrel on the bird table was still nibbling away hungrily.
9.27 a.m.	I sipped de-caf coffee, and nibbled one of the last two Black Magic chocolates, the Raspberry Parfait. Mmmm.. ....it's what's inside that's special. Mmmm..... must write to pen-friends, my aunt and niece.
9.51 a.m.	Purrdita and Cleopatra, curled up either side of me on the sofa, purring softly, while I picked up a pen. I like having a cat either side of me, because cats are like chocolates, it's hard to have just ....
9.52 a.m.	I wrote a short letter to my niece, in a card I knew she would *love*; a painting of baby owls sitting in a row (all fluffy feathers and bright eyes) by the wonderful wild- life artist, Pollyanna Pickering. When I had stamped and addressed the envelope, I enjoyed sticking an owl opposite the stamp, an autumn leaf, then a rabbit, because Louise loves rabbits too.

10.10 a.m.	Nibbled on an Orange Sensation chocolate, because like cats, it's hard to have just ......
10.13 a.m.	The magical dark treat perked up my brain, ready to write three little notes in wildlife cards, to my aunt and pen-friends. I had fun sicking hedgehogs, colourful leaves, trees, and pine cones on the envelopes. Then smiled, admiring my hard day's work.

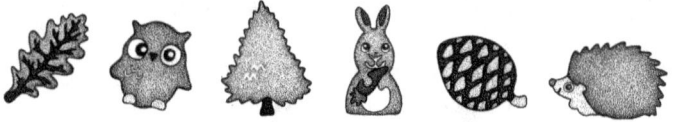

11.35 a.m.	Joe Browns catalogue arrived with the post. I always smile when I flick through their pages of *cool funky fashions*; great gifts for my teenage niece and nephew, and Ben. He likes to wear their flamboyant shirts to birthday parties, and his Avocado Pair gigs. I wear their black leggings; very good quality. Leggings from some other catalogues are as thin as toilet paper, and only fit for an anorexic giraffe to wear.
12.05 p.m.	I think I will order the Barcelona shirt for Ben. It's a charismatic stripe shirt; confident, offbeat, and self assured. It will suit Ben *perfectly*, it's his birthday soon.
12.09 p.m.	A funky cat flap? I didn't know Joe Browns sold pet goods!
12.10 p.m.	Oh, funky flat cap. I must have my M.E. eyeballs in today.
12.12 p.m.	The Fender tee-shirt looks *just right* for my nephew, who loves to play electric guitar. My niece will like the jumper with big red hearts, because she loved the heart jewellery I gave her last Christmas from Joe Browns.
12.14 p.m.	The Crazy Alpine Leggings look really *cool*. A deranged avalanche of colours; mustard and brown, red and turquoise stripes, white alpine designs. I'm *so* tempted to order a pair for myself, to liven up my tired old legs. Shall I order them?

I don't *really* need new leggings, I have plenty of black pairs. But I do *love* the avalanche of deranged colours, *and* red is an energy giving colour. So is turquoise. They are quite pricey, five pounds more than the black leggings. They are *very unusual* though, and I think my legs would like a change after nearly twenty years of living in black leggings. I *do* like stripes. The mustard and brown stripes are very autumnal, and the little white alpine designs are *so sweet*. Oh, why not, what the hell! When you have M.E. you will do anything to give you a little energy and brighten your life, if you can afford a little luxury.

Ever notice that 'what the hell' is always the right decision?

MARILYN MONROE

12.30 p.m.   There's a half price sale in today's ACE catalogue. I like the bird wall art. If the birds were seagulls, they would look wonderful in my house on the Cornish coast, next door to Dawn French. I do enjoy a peaceful living-by-the-sea daydream.

12.35 p.m.   I'm awoken from my daydream by the wind, making the windows rattle, and whistling through the gaps in the back door.

12.36 p.m.   Leaves are flying across the lawn; they look like yellow, green and brown birds. I've been dreaming about bird jigsaw puzzles; the birds fly out of the puzzle, leaving just a blue sky. Then I grow wings, and fly out of the window with the birds.

Dreaming permits each and every one of us to be quietly and safely insane every night of our lives

CHARLES WILLIAM DEMENT

Saturday 16th

When I fed our wildlife, first thing this morning, I was showered with a flurry of sycamore leaves. A large one rested on my chest, like the gentle hand of a healer. I thought about the healing power of nature, and for a moment, I came over all poetic.

AUTUMN LEAF

An autumn leaf
Upon my chest
Mother nature
Knows what's best

Then I noticed I had a leaf stuck in my hair. I thought about hedgehogs hibernating under leaves, and suddenly, as the cold made me shiver, I felt the urge to hibernate in bed for the winter. I plodded back indoors, with another verse in my head.

AUTUMN LEAVES

Autumn is falling
Onto my head
Now it's time
I was tucked up
In bed

I thought it would be a *very good* idea to take a supply of chocolate to bed with me, when I hibernated for the winter. A large tin of Quality Street, Roses chocolates, After Eight minty chocs, and a *whole* **Death by Chocolate** cake, would be *perfect*. I fell back into bed with more verse in my head.

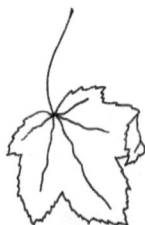

DEATH BY CHOCOLATE

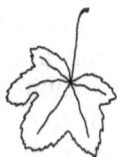

Like
Autumn
Leaves
Falling
Out
Of
The
Sky
Sometimes
I Want
To
Just
Curl
Up
And
Die
A
Death
By
Chocolate
Is
Just
What
I
Need
I'll
Lie
Under
The
Covers
And
Constantly
Feed

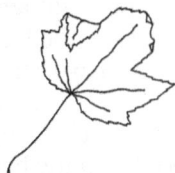

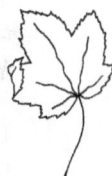

I
Like
Autumn
Leaves
Falling
Out
Of
The
Sky

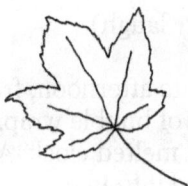

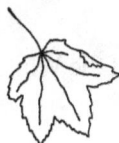

I
Like
Autumn
Leaves
Falling

Fortunately I awoke late afternoon feeling a lot more cheerful, less fatigued and weary. My autumn edition of M.E. Essential magazine was waiting for me, and I enjoyed a good read. I particularly liked the photographs of a little art exhibition, held in a vegetarian café in Oxford, the Magic Café. The exhibition was called, What is M.E.? And all the artwork and photos were by people who have M.E.

The witch in my book is a vegetarian, and would like the Magic Café. I would love to have attended the exhibition, and written about it in my book. I especially liked Comfort Blanket; a painting of a girl in bed, her blanket, a collage of supplements and pill packets. I found it *so moving*, the image will stay in my memory for always. Or as long as my leaky cauldron head will allow.

When Ben arrived home from a trip to Sainsbury's and Holland & Barrett, I showed him the article.

ME: This exhibition looked good.

BEN: Yes dear.

ME: I would like a small exhibition of my work and an ex-boyfriend named Hibition. Then I could introduce him to everyone as my ex Hibition.

BEN: Most amusing *dear* (Basil Fawlty laugh).

My dad's birthday gift arrived late afternoon, from Scots of Stow catalogue, well wrapped in a blanket of bubble wrap. It was a clock. But no ordinary clock, a *most unusual* melted clock. A homage to the wonderful artist Salvador Dali. I showed it to Ben.

ME: This is wonderfully surreal isn't it?
                Looks just like the clocks, or watches, in Dali's paintings.

BEN: *Absolutely* dear.

ME: I feel inspired to complete more of the White Rabbit's watch in my Disney puzzle.

BEN: That's marvellous, but now I'm late for a *very important date, no time to say hello, goodbye......*

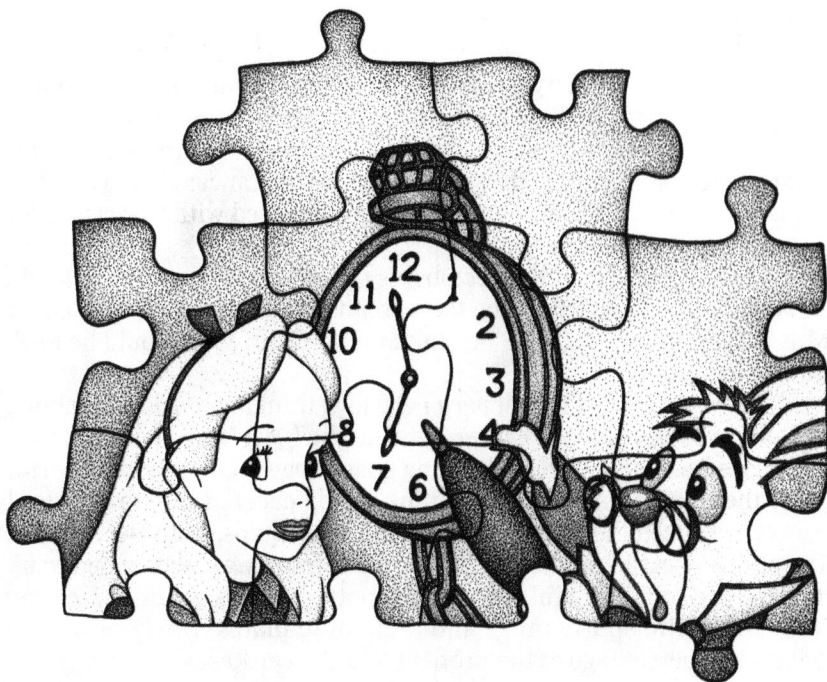

ME: Very amusing *dear* (Basil Fawlty's wife's voice).

* * * * * *

After I had fished around for a while in a sea of puzzle pieces, my head began to swim a little; but I managed to piece together the watch, part of Alice, and the White Rabbit. As I started to tire Cleopatra came to the rescue again. She climbed into the puzzle box and passed wind. I imagined the little Disney characters holding their noses; Grumpy grumbling, Happy laughing, and Sneezy sneezing. When she fell asleep, I wondered if cats had surreal dreams.

Although I had slept a lot the night before, I wanted to curl up in the puzzle box and dream Disney dreams all winter. I'm looking forward to when our little town becomes a silent winter wonderland, under a thick snow white blanket.

Sunday 17th

I read in Weekly Wife, that one in nine British women will be diagnosed with breast cancer during their lifetime. Breast cancer is the most common type of cancer in the UK, and more than 45,000 women and 250 men, are diagnosed with breast cancer every year. But the good news is, eight out of ten women diagnosed with breast cancer, now survive beyond five years.

I also read that October is breast cancer awareness month, and was a little shocked by the facts about the disease. I thought about M.E. awareness week (the 8th to 14th May). I think May should be M.E. awareness month.

I started to feel *very very* low, thinking of friends, family, and pets who have died of cancer. What a *cruel cruel* monster. I can't say any more dear diary, I'll make your pages soggy. On a more cheerful note, the double-page spread of pink goods cheered me up a little. I particularly liked the pink heart cushion with sequins, from Debenhams. The pink pomegranate and elderflower juice, from www.bottlegreen.co.uk looked nice too. The pink and white spotty glasses would match my pink and white spotty mugs and melamine plates. I may order the glasses — a percentage of the profits go to Cancer Research.

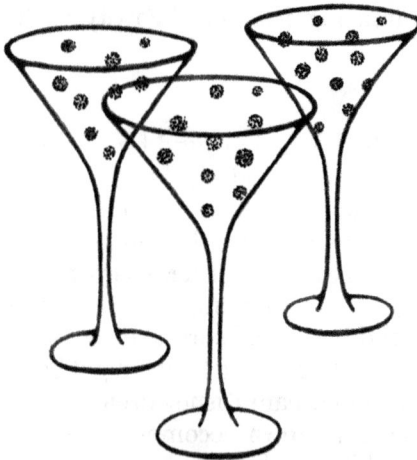

3.00 p.m. A text message from Jayne:

HI WITCHY FRIEND, I-M STARTING TO GET DREAM
PREMONITIONS AGAIN, AS I-M DOING TAROT READINGS
REGULARLY NOW - I DREAMT THAT SUMTHIN TO DO WITH UR
HEALTH IS WORRYING YOU - SLEEPY HUGS X X X

3.01 p.m. I thought I would reply to Jayne, telling her I was a little
concerned about having a mammogram, because alternative
medicine has maintained for years that mammograms can
do more harm than good. Their ionising radiation mutates
cells, and the mechanical pressure on the breast can spread
cells that are already malignant.
Ben found out about thermography on the internet.
Mammography cannot detect a tumour until it has been
growing for years and reaches a certain size. Thermography
can detect the possibility of cancer much earlier, because
it can image the early stages of increased blood supply to
cancer cells, which is a necessary step, before they can grow
into a detectable sized tumour. An infra red camera detects
the heat (infra red radiation) which is emitted by the breast
without physical contact (no compression) and without
sending any signal (no radiation).
There's a hospital, only forty minutes drive away in
Tunbridge Wells, that will do this type of breast scan. It
sounds *much* safer.

* * * * * * *

I decided to send a short text message to Jayne, a *com-
pressed* version of the information, but it took me a while to remember
the word thermography. The first word that came to mind was theology,
then trigonometry.

3.03 p.m. Geography..... No..... Triathlon..... No..... Trecastle.....
Trefeitha..... No, Welsh villages..... thermometer.....
thermology.

3.04 p.m. Thermography, hurrah!

3.05 p.m.   Brain so foggy and tired from the effort of word search, I'm tempted to send crazy text message:

HI TAROT READING WITCH, I-M WORRIED ABOUT A MAMMOTH – BUT I WILL TRY TRIGONOMETRY INSTEAD – HAPPY HUGS X

Or:

HI, I WAS A WOOLY MAMMOTH ONCE – NOW I-M A TIRANOSAURUS REX – HEDGE HOGS X

3.07 p.m.   Sent a text message:

HI TAROT WITCH, U R RIGHT – I-M A BIT WORRIED ABOUT MAMMOGRAM – GONNA TRY THERMOGRAPHY – IT SOUNDS SAFER – WARM HUG X

3.20 p.m.   Noticed the wildlife in our garden needed more peanuts, and as I plodded outside an aeroplane flew quite low overhead. A few lines of verse popped into my head. Not my verse. A certain singer I've been listening to.

Daniel is travelling
Tonight on a plane
I can see the red tail lights
Heading for Spain.....

3.21 p.m.   Wondered if the plane *was* heading for Spain.

3.45 p.m.   In bath, listening to a CD.

She packed my bags
Last night preflight
Zero hour nine a.m.
And I'm gonna be high
As a kite by then

3.47 p.m.   Singing to self.

And I think it's gonna be

115

A long long time
La la la la la
La la la la la
La la la la la
La la la la la
Oh, no no no
I'm a rocket man
Ooooooooh! ROCKET MAN!
La la la la la up here alone

4.00 p.m.   *When are you gonna come down*
When are you going to land
La la la   la la la.....

4.02 p.m.   The witch in my book prefers to fly to Scotland on a plane, rather than on her broomstick. I used to fly by aeroplane to Scotland with easyJet. I should have had my witch flying by easyBroom.

4.03 p.m.   No, *no, no, no*. I'm not having these thoughts any more. The book is done, done, done. *Completely* completed. *Perfectly* printed. I wonder when I will hear from A.F.M.E.

4.04 p.m.   I have a feeling it will be soon, easyBroomsticks crossed!

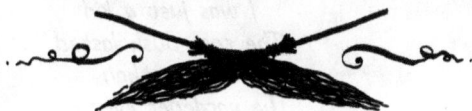

4.20 p.m.   Watched the rain wash away the petals of the last rose in our garden.

4.21 p.m.   Felt a little sad.

4.22 p.m.   Wrote a song in my head, to the tune of Elton's, *Candle in the Wind*.

MARILYN MONROSE

Goodbye Marilyn
I planted you, and you grew tall
With grace to hold yourself
While creepy crawlies crawled
They crawled up your woodwork
From the lawn they'd start
And it breaks heart
Watching your blooms disappear
As your petals fall apart

And it seems to me
You lived your life
Like a petal in the wind
Never knowing
Where to cling to
When the rain set in

For many years
I've grown you
I was just a kid
The rose bush lasted
Longer than
The gardener ever did

Chapter
Three

October

Monday 18th

Charles William Dement was *so* right when he said that dreaming permits us to be quietly insane every night. Last night I dreamt I was cooking a Disney jigsaw puzzle in a big black cauldron. *Cooking a jigsaw puzzle!*

As I added witchy ingredients to create bright colours: turmeric (for yellow), onion skin (for orange), madder root (for red), blueberries (for blue), coltsfoot and bracken (for green); Disney characters appeared, swirling in the steam. Peter Pan flew around with Tinkerbell and Aladdin followed them on a magic carpet.

Maybe this is how witches do their jigsaw puzzles. They pour the puzzle pieces into a cauldron of water, boil them up with plant dyes, then watch colourful images emerge. Sounds like a good idea to me. More fun than the normal way, and your neck doesn't seize up.

I completed the Peter Pan part of my puzzle. He looked great, full of life and joy, flying through the air with his arms outstretched. His clothes were very green, like leaves. My neck didn't feel so great. Very stiff, like a tree trunk. My face looked a little green, like a tired old witch; and the only thing flying through the air was cat hairs, as I stroked Cleopatra's silky coat.

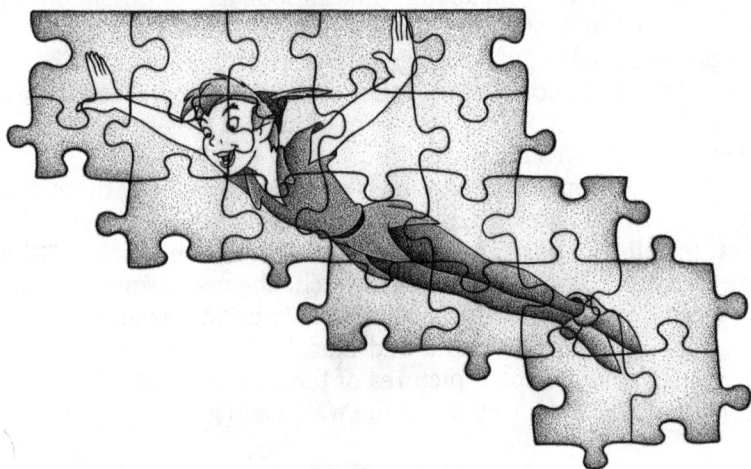

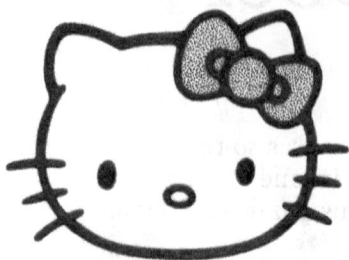

I was snowed under with Christmas gift catalogues today, so I wrapped my neck in a warm towel and lay on the sofa for a sleepy browse. I spotted a few stocking fillers for my niece; the Santa chocolate jigsaw puzzle, reindeer droppings (caramel) and snowman droppings (mint imperials) looked sweet. I wondered if Louise would like the Hello Kitty or Betty Boop fragrances, and was tempted to order the Hello Kitty watch for myself — the strap on my old one is falling apart. I need a new alarm clock too.

The Hello Kitty alarm clock set looked good. Very pink. Very girly. *And* you get a watch to match. Also the Hello Kitty jigsaw puzzle was delightful. If I had a watch and alarm clock to match, I could time how long it took me to complete parts of the puzzle. A new hobby.

I liked the Betty Boop pyjamas and hot water bottle, with an alarm clock to match. I'm tempted by the Betty Boop gifts because I love my Betty Boop socks; soft ice-cream colours, with humorous pictures of Betty. They make me smile as soon as I put them on. Most of my socks are looking rather sad and old. Many have pictures of frogs or Tigger, and used to put a spring in my step for five seconds. They look like they have M.E. now, because they are worn, a little threadbare and the colours are faded. Betty puts some colour and life back into my sock drawer, and she gives me happy feet.

She must be very busy promoting herself, there are so many Betty ornaments; a table lamp, make-up set, weekend bag and wallet, jewellery hanger..... I couldn't see a watch, but I spotted a Disney fairy one. It was a Tinkerbell watch. She had turquoise wings, a leafy green dress and pom-pom slippers. My mind was made up.

Hannah Montana had many gifts in her name too. My niece used to like Hannah, pictures of the star adorned her bedroom wall. I wondered if she would like the watch and gift set.

| 3.05 p.m. | Sent a text message: |

HI SIS, I-M ORDERIN XMAS GIFTS – DUZ LOU STILL LIKE HANNAH MONTANA?

| 6.07 p.m. | Ben came home from work. |

| ME: | We're having deep Peter Pan pizza for dinner. |

| BEN: | *Marvellous* dear, are there Tinkerbell fairy cakes too? |

Tuesday 19th

I spent the night finishing my Disney puzzle on the lawn. The puzzle pieces were paper thin, and when an October breeze blew across the lawn, they were tossed into the air with autumn leaves, and turned into butterflies, all the colours of the rainbow. They flew away with Tinkerbell, her little turquoise wings fluttering madly. I woke up scatter-brained, with fluttery eyelashes.

I day dreamt of having a lovely pair of turquoise wings, and being able to flutter about all day. I imagined going to the doctor, suffering from wing flop, I smiled, then I fell back to sleep. I dreamt I wore pink Betty Boop pyjamas, and all the little Bettys were fluttering their eyelashes. Then they turned into frogs and Tiggers, hopping and bouncing onto the bed.

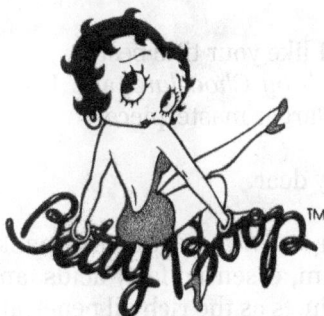

I didn't feel very bouncy when I awoke, nor did I feel the urge to continue with my puzzle, because my neck was still seized up from yesterday's efforts. Instead I leafed through my *M.E. Essential* again, and felt inspired to create my *own* Comfort Blanket artwork. Decided to call my masterpiece, *Death by Chocolate*, and found the chocolate wrappers I had saved. I wrapped my neck in a warm towel, drew a quick sketch of myself sleeping under a quilt in an A4 sketchpad, then cut the wrappers into little squares to make a colourful quilt cover. When I had glued the squares *artily* onto my drawing, I imagined creating the picture much larger, with After Eight choc wrapper squares, for some dark contrast.

Before Ben drove into town to do his weekly Avocado Pair gig, I showed him *Death by Chocolate*.

ME: What do you think?

BEN: Very nice dear.

ME: Can you guess the title?

BEN: Quality sleep time?

ME: Very good, but no.

BEN: Sweet dreams?

ME: Cackle, cackle!

BEN: Yes?

ME: No, but I like your title best.
           It's *Death by Chocolate*, and I need more chocolate to create a larger masterpiece.

BEN: Certainly dear.

ME: Did you know avocados are packed with vitamin E, potassium, essential fatty acids, and are often found in spa products as the rich oil penetrates into the skin?

BEN: *Fascinating* dear.

ME: I must put some on the shopping list, the oil promotes a radiant complexion.

BEN: Will I come home to find you with mashed avocado all over your face?

ME: Probably.

Wednesday 20th

Ben has composed some *wonderfully witchy* music for my website, advertising *Love & Best Witches*. Also, a friend at his works has been helping us with the site. You can turn over pages of extracts from the book when you visit the site, and we wanted a magical tinkly sound as the pages turn.

10.29 a.m.   Text message from Ben:

> STEVE HAS DONE A BRILL JOB ON NEW VERSION OF FLIPP IN PAGE-BOOK FOR WEBSITE – HE-S JUST GOT TO ADD WITCHY TINKLE SOUND WHEN THE PAGES TURN – IT LOOKS HEAPS BETTER, REALLY PRO X

10.30 a.m.   I replied:

> THAT-S GREAT NEWS – WILL SIGN A COPY OF MY BOOK FOR STEVE X

11.05 a.m.   Text message from my sister:

> HI, CONGRATS ON YOR BOOK – IT LOOKS GREAT – LOU HAS SNAFFLED IT AWAY SO I DIDN-T C IT 4 LONG – LOU LIKES HANNAH BUT NOT CLOTHES WITH HER ON X

11.06 a.m.   I replied:

> THANKS SIS – WILL SEND A COPY OF MY BOOK 4 U X

11.08 a.m.   I sent Jayne a text message:

HI TAROT-WITCH, WEBSITE IS LOOKIN BETTER – CHECK IT OUT
WHEN U CAN X V X

11.10 a.m.   Jayne replied:

OH, THAT-S WONDERFUL WITCHY NEWS X

Mid-afternoon a large parcel arrived by courier. It was big enough to hold six telephone directories, or those enormous Next catalogues. Before I opened it, I tried to think what the contents might be, I didn't have a clue. What had I ordered recently? I knew a couple of calendars, and a pack of Christmas cards were due to arrive from the R.N.L.I., because I'd written a reminder on my calendar. The box was very light, hardly weighed a thing, so it didn't hold six telephone directories. Two calendars and a pack of cards would be a small flat package.

When I opened the box I was still flummoxed, it was full of giant bubble wrap, each bubble almost the size of a house brick. I pulled out the sheets of AIRplus bubbles, and there, at the bottom of the box, were two calendars and a pack of Christmas cards from the R.N.L.I. I laughed, no, I *cackled*, because the bubble wrap reminded me of life jackets. If the box had been lost overboard at sea, it would have floated happily to shore, like a message in a bottle.

Sometimes I receive gifts from catalogues that are not packaged well enough, and arrive damaged. The R.N.L.I. *certainly* know how to ensure their goods arrive safely. On dry land.

There was an R.N.L.I. gift catalogue in the box with my goods; all sorts of gifts that would look *simply wonderful* in my beach house on the Cornish coast, next door to Dawn French. I liked the seagull wall art (although I don't think the artist has ever seen a seagull), the beach hut doorstop, and beach hut cushion.

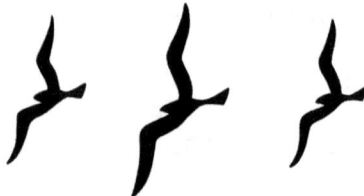

In my mind's eye I could see, in my kitchen; the stripy Sail-away mugs with a teapot, milk jug, and Port and Starboard egg cups to match. *And* I could clearly visualise myself wearing the Nautical but Nice apron, as I stood at my kitchen sink doing the washing-up, watching Dawn French picking up a message in a bottle, washed-up on her private beach.

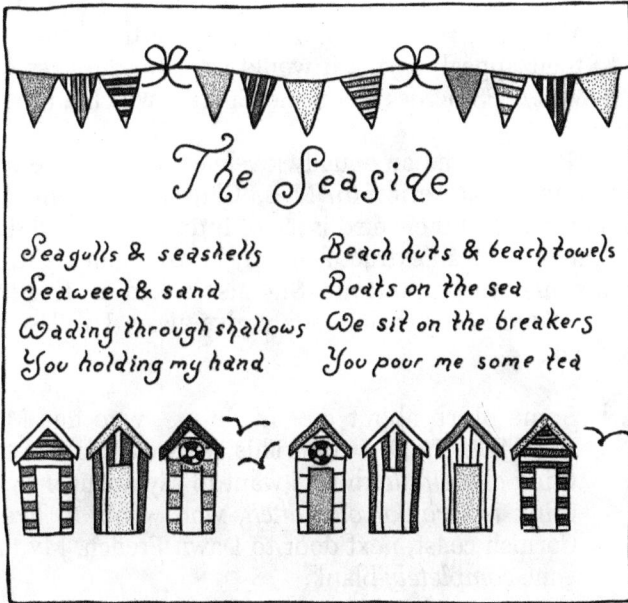

The Seaside

Seagulls & seashells
Seaweed & sand
Wading through shallows
You holding my hand

Beach huts & beach towels
Boats on the sea
We sit on the breakers
You pour me some tea

This week's kitchen roll design would be perfect for my beach house too. It's a bright red, white and navy blue design, with beach huts and bunting. As I tore off a sheet to blow my nose, I daydreamt of spending a day at the seaside, the bracing sea breeze blowing away my M.E. brain fog. But at this time of year, I didn't fancy shivering on a deserted pebbly beach, freezing my nose off. So I did the next best thing. I imagined Ben and I sitting on the breakers at Whitstable, staring out to sea, as we munched egg and cress sandwiches, and sipped tea from a flask. Then I wrote some verse on a handy piece of seaside kitchen roll. Because that's what kitchen roll is for, blowing your nose and writing poetry.

I don't think the artist who designed the kitchen roll has ever seen a seagull either. But it really doesn't matter, the whole drawing is lovely. I can almost hear the seagulls calling, the bunting flapping in a sea breeze, and waves splashing onto the shore.

Thursday 21st

Today I received a letter from the Chairman of the Kent and Sussex M.E./CFS society, Colin Barton. He thanked me for my donation to their appeal; saying it would improve the lives of people affected by M.E./CFS across Kent and Sussex, which I thought was *really nice.*

Ben received an equally lovely email from the press and publications officer at Action for M.E., Clare Ogden. She said they were planning pages of their next issue of Inter Action, and thought it would be grand to use an extract from my book, about eight hundred words, and some blurb about me. She also asked for five copies of *Love & Best Witches*, for their readers give-away. I will send seven copies. For luck.

6.30 p.m.   Some blurb about *me!* Little *me*, who has M.E. In a *MAGAZINE!* Oh God. This is wonderful, but I can't think of a *single* thing I want to say about *me*. All I can think is; *cranky old witch*, who wants to live on the Cornish coast, next door to Dawn French. My mind has gone *completely* blank.

6.35 p.m.   I still don't know what to write.

6.37 p.m.   Maybe I'll have some coffee and plain chocolate to perk up my sleepy brain; it's just sitting in my skull, like a hibernating tortoise in a box, in granny's old wardrobe.

6.44 p.m.   *The tortoise has woken up, blinked his eyes and shuffled around in the box.*

6.45 p.m.   Have written a few lines, but recalling past years of coping with M.E. is making me feel a little tearful.

6.48 p.m.	Cross out what I've written, it all reads a bit miserable. Will start again.
6.49 p.m.	*The tortoise wipes away a tear on his comfortable bedding and feels a little peckish.*
6.50 p.m.	Nibble two more squares of plain choc.
7.14 p.m.	Hurrah! have written four *whole* paragraphs.
7.15 p.m.	Cross out paragraphs, they *still* read a little too gloomy. I need to be more concise.
7.41 p.m.	Have written five short paragraphs. Much better. Brain *very* tired.
7.42 p.m.	*The tortoise is tempted to go back into hibernation.*
8.05 p.m.	Leaf through *Love & Best Witches*, while I nibble on an After Eight choc, trying to decide which extracts to use.
8.06 p.m.	*The tortoise nibbles on a leaf and decides not to go back into hibernation just yet.*
8.07 p.m.	I can't decide which extracts to use. Maybe the paragraph on page 38 about chocolate loving fairies. No. Or, the healing spell on page 114. Possibly. The Mary Poppins spell on page 107? No. The making of a witch's wand, and taking cauldrons of soup to people who are bedridden with M.E. on page 58. Yes, I'm *almost* certain. Must count the words in the paragraphs. Maybe I'll include a poem.
8.15 p.m.	Have counted words in seven paragraphs and poems. I keep losing count. Brain falling asleep. Neck seizing up. 446 words so far.
8.18 p.m.	Must have no more than 800 words. I quite like the section about making Harry Potter chocolate frog cookies. They add

up to 200 words. That's too many because I want to use several extracts.

8.20 p.m.   I'm going cross-eyed with a witchy squint.

8.21 p.m.   Cleopatra sits on the book; it's a good excuse for me to rest, I'm starting a headache and my neck hurts. Feel like I've counted 8 million words, lost count 8 thousand times, and changed my mind 8 hundred times.

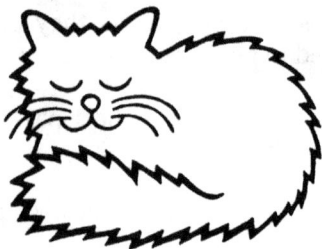

8.22 p.m.   Lying on bed, massaging neck with eyes closed. *Oh God!* Why did I write this silly book about a barmy old witch, feeding whisky to dragons and chocolate to fairies. *Why!* Nobody will want to read it, and I'm really not sure about any of the extracts I've chosen.

8.24 p.m.   I must be a more confident and decisive author, with a professional attitude.

8.25 p.m.   Feel like drinking a few glasses of beautiful deep red Merlot to ease my fatigue. Passing out. Then waking up, with face stuck to beautiful deep blue shiny cover of book, to find the beautiful pink book fairies have made all the decisions for me.

8.26 p.m.   *Not* a very professional attitude.

9.30 p.m.   Will not drink wine.
             Will eat choc instead.

9.31 p.m.   Gently remove big hairy cat bum from the copy of *Love & Best Witches*. Cleopatra passes wind to show her displeasure, she was having such magical feline dreams about riding with me on my broomstick. I sneeze.

9.32 p.m.   I blow my nose on seaside kitchen roll.

9.46 p.m.   Maybe I'll use the extract about a healing spell for a cold on page 94. No. I think I prefer the spell on page 137, and it's 108 words. I like the section about reading the tea leaves too, only 102 words. The paragraph about the wizardly boots is nice and short, and makes me smile:

I noticed a pair of wizardly boots by auntie's back door. I asked her who they belonged to, and her face went as red as her strawberry jam. She said a wizard friend had given them to her for gardening. But auntie doesn't have the energy to do any gardening!

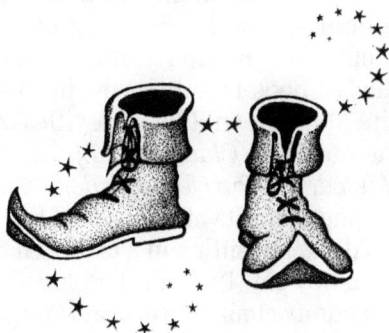

9.48 p.m.   I think it would be a good final extract, although I'm not *completely* sure. I must decide. Must be more *decisive*. It's 50 words, and brings the total number of words to 752. I like that number. A good number.

9.49 p.m.   Yes, I think I've *actually* made up my mind.
              752 sounds just right. *Perfect.*

10.30 p.m.	In bed. Dreaming about wizards and love. And best witches. And living on the Cornish coast, in a wonderful beach house, with my own private beach, next door to Dawn French. Loving best beaches.
10.31 p.m.	*The tortoise closes his weary eyes, and dreams he is a turtle, drifting into the deep green seas of hibernation.*

Friday 22nd

6.10 p.m.	Ben arrived home from work. Took off shoes. Checked emails.
6.11 p.m.	WOW! *Witchily wonderful!* A.F.M.E. Have decided to do a double-page spread, and would like a photo of me to go with the short biography and extracts. I will have to see if I can find one, I've rarely had my photo taken since I got ill. But there will be a few, taken at home with my cats. I'm not going to do one of those *author at desk* poses, looking intelligent and writerly, with pen poised or book in hand. I never sit at a desk anyway. Or look intelligent. Or writerly. But pale and witchy, yes.

The last book I read was by the fabulous American writer, Rita Mae Brown. I love the titles of her books: *Murder – She Meowed, Claws and Effect, Puss 'n Cahoots, Santa Clawed, The Purrfect Murder*; to name, only a few. There is a photo of Rita at the back of her book. She is not posing at a desk, but sitting in a comfy chair looking tranquil with her tabby cat. I will find a photo of me looking tranquil. In a comfy chair. With a cat. *Purrfect.*

6.20 p.m.	Find photos taken over the past few years. There's me in bed with cats draped around my neck, like a colourful furry scarf. One of me lying on the sofa at Christmas, ginger paper hat and cat to match. Sitting on the lawn in the summer, surrounded by cats. Asleep in chair with grey cat. Sitting on sofa at Halloween, wearing pointy black hat, with black cat on lap. Lying on sofa, under a furry blanket of cats.

6.30 p.m.   The photo taken last Halloween, with my black cat, will be ideal for promoting a witchy book. There's a new tartan rug on the sofa too, which will be apt, because there's a lot of *Scottish-ness* in my book, with Nessie and Loch Ness, and a Scottish dragon.

7.00 p.m.   In kitchen serving up dinner. Smiling as I put a double dollop of coleslaw on Ben's baked potato.

7.01 p.m.   A *double-page spread!* Little people like me don't get double-page spreads. Maybe a slice of Sara Lee *double* chocolate gateaux, or *double* cream on a mince pie at Christmas. Or *double* crème fraîche topping on a Soignon goats cheese and spinach tart, or *double* Gloucester cheese on a cream cracker, Boxing Day. Or a *double chocolate sundae* on a Sunday.

8.00 p.m.   In bath. Smiling.
Little people like me, are lucky to get a *double* six when we play Monopoly, so our boot can pass go and collect 200 pounds. Maybe, on our birthday, receive a box of Thornton's chocolates; creamy truffles, light mousses and smooth pralines, covered in rich dark chocolate, with a *double* layer. Or indulge in *double* helpings of choc chip ice cream on a hot summer's day.

9.00 p.m.   Watching TV. Smiling.
Little witches like me, are lucky to be able to enjoy a *double* bill of our favourite spooky, period drama, or a good *double* agent film.

11.00 p.m. Getting undressed for bed. Smiling.
Little witchy people like me, are lucky to get *double* ruff cuffs, and a *double* ribbed hem on a lightweight knit dress, or a *double*-breasted trench coat with shimmering fabric. But never a *DOUBLE-PAGE SPREAD*.

Saturday 23rd

12.35 p.m.   Text message from my sister:

THANK U V MUCH 4 THE BOOK - TOOK LOU SHOPPIN 2DAY -
SHE IS SIZE 14 - GETTIN TALLER - MORE TEENAGE -
CONGRATS ON DOUBLE PAGE SPREAD X

1.05 p.m.   Text message from Jayne:

OH, THAT-S WONDERFUL NEWS ABOUT THE DOUBLE PAGE
SPREAD - HAPPY WITCH HUG X

1.30 p.m.   Text message from Ben:

I-M IN SAINS-B, LET ME KNOW IF THERE-S ANY TREATS YOU-
D LIKE X

1.31 p.m.   I reply:

DIVINE CHOC BAR - JAR OF DOUBLE PAGE SPREAD - HAHAHA
- THANX X

1.33 p.m.   Enjoy a delicious daydream. Sitting on the veranda of my
dream home by the sea, next door to Dawn French, reading
a fabulous review of my latest novel. Sipping champagne
and nibbling Divine chocolate, which really *is* divine.

I text Dawn to tell her my good news and she replies:

HI, CONGRATS - WILL POP ROUND TO CELEBRATE LATER -
MAYBE U COULD WRITE A SKETCH FOR MY NEW TV SHOW -
DAWN X

I reply:

OH YES - THAT WUD BE GREAT - ABSOLUTELY FABULOUS -
SEE U LATER - VERITY X

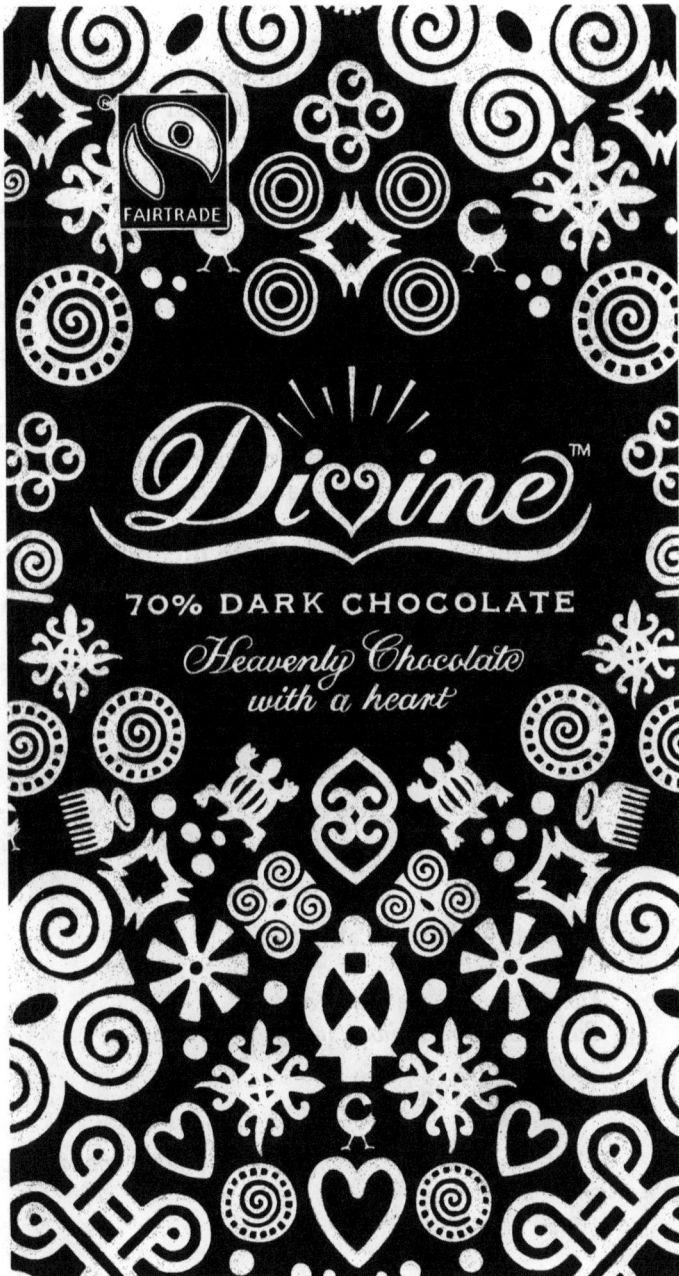

Sunday 24th

It was such a beautiful autumn day today, I smiled as brightly as sunshine on a bald man's head, when I put food out for the wildlife. I don't know why I thought of a bald man's head. Maybe it's because Ben likes me to put suntan lotion on his bald patch (on a hot day) and we were laughing about it last night — I call it his crop circle.

The air was cold, fresh and happy; happy as a little person who is looking forward to her very own *double-page spread*. I couldn't believe how well I felt, and I was even a little energetic. Well, just a little, and just a little is *a lot* when you have M.E.

As I ate breakfast, I daydreamed about writing a sketch about chocolate with Dawn French, in my home on the Cornish Coast. We would have to eat lots of chocolates, chocolate gateaux and biscuits and puddings for a week, for research. I'm sure Dawn wouldn't mind. Maybe we could do a chocolate jigsaw puzzle, and when we had completed it (weeks later) celebrate the success of our **whole show about chocolate**, by eating it *and* a **whole box** of Belgian Guylian chocolate shells. I wonder if a lot of writers love chocolate, I know Roald Dahl does:

> *Never mind about 1066 William the Conqueror, 1087 William the second. Such things are not going to affect one's life.....*
> *But 1932 Mars Bar and 1936 Maltesers and 1937 Kit~Kat ~ these are milestones in history and should be seared into the memory of every child in the country.*

And Patrick Skene Catling:

> *Other things are just food.*
> *But chocolate's chocolate.*

And Judith Olney:

> *Most chocolate chip cookies do not have enough chocolate chips in them.*

After breakfast I was very tempted to do lots of chores. But I was strong, and I thought, no. *NO. NO. NO.* I needed to conserve my energy, my precious small amount of energy, for my afternoon out on Tuesday. It's Ben's birthday on the 26th, and I *LOVE* to celebrate with him.

He visited his best friend Bill, for a pre-birthday celebration today. Bill has recently moved to Hastings Old Town, near the fishermen's huts. He is an artist, and living near the seaside is ideal for his painting. Living on the Cornish coast would be ideal for my writing.

Before Ben went out, he printed off the extracts and brief biog about me for A.F.M.E., so I could check for mistakes. The pages were waiting for me next to his computer, when I emerged from a midday nap.

2.00 p.m.   I sent Ben a text message:

THANX 4 FAB TYPING - GIV OLD BILL MY LUV X

2.05 p.m.   Ben replied:

OLD BILL SENDS HIS LUV - WALKIN ON BEACH - SUNNY BUT V CHILLY X

3.05 p.m.   I continued to rest and ignored the urge to clean the cooker, and the bathroom and..... and.....

3.06 p.m   My cats inspired me to keep resting. Mary lay soaking up the afternoon sun in the window. Cleopatra was in her favourite place, on our printer; she's part of the family now. Purrdita snored in her favourite chair, paws and whiskers twitching.

8.00 p.m.   After dinner I watched the Antiques Roadshow. There were some items belonging to writer, Agatha Christie. I wondered if she'd ever had a *double-page spread.* Or loved chocolate. Or both.

8.01 p.m.   Recalled reading an article about Agatha Christie once. Was it a double-page spread? I don't know. Anyway, it quoted her saying that there's nothing like boredom to make you write. I can SO identify with that.

8.02 p.m.   Agatha's second marriage was to an archaeologist, and she wrote many of her mystery stories as she accompanied him on various digs around the world. She once said, 'An archaeologist is the best husband a woman can have. The older she gets the more interested he is in her.'

8.03 p.m.   Agatha was a wise woman. I wonder if Ben has ever thought of taking up archaeology as a hobby.

8.04 p.m.   A-r-c-h-a-e-o-l-o-g-y. Hmm. That's a word I have to think about before I write it down. If you are a witch who can spell archaeology, archaeologist or archaeological, without thinking too much, or consulting your Oxford English mini dictionary (Hmm, lets see... *ah*, page 25... archipelago... architect... architrave... no *ologists* on this page... how about page 24... archetype... archdeacon... archbishop... archangel... Ahah! archaeology... I *knew* there was an *a* before the *eo*... I'd just forgotten) then you are a witch who is really good at *spelling*.

8.05 p.m.   Text message from Ben:

HAVIN A DRINK IN THE MERMAID IN RYE X

8.06 p.m   I replied:

IN THE 18ᵀᴴ CENTURY, SMUGGLERS MET IN THAT PUB, SMOKING PIPES, WITH LOADED PISTOLS ON THEIR TABLES – THE INFAMOUS HAWKHURST GANG – A MURDEROUS LOT

8.08 p.m.   Ben replied:

FASCINATING DEAR

8.10 p.m.   In a silly mood, I had to send another message:

YES, HISTORY IS INTERESTING, HAV YOU EVER THORT OF TAKING UP ARCHAEOLOGY?

8.12 p.m.   WHAT R U LIKE?

8.15 p.m.   Decided to find more of the Little Mermaid in my Disney puzzle, and encourage Ben to take up archaeology. I used to belong to the Sittingbourne and Swale Archaeological Research Group. I loved going on digs and drawing the pottery finds. I will tell Ben *all* about it, and encourage him to watch Time Team on Channel 4, with the wonderful Tony Robinson. This week the team will be excavating a site in North Wales, which may date back to the Iron Age. It's quite exciting, once you get into the programme. Tony's team are *so enthusiastic,* especially when they find a skeleton! Last week, they found the skeleton of a small nun (probably in her thirties) in a Saxon monastery burial ground. When Tony exclaimed, what a lovely set of teeth she had (and what good condition her bones were in) I imagined her having a giggle in spirit world. Every girl likes to feel attractive. She may have been considered quite plain in her day, and now, *at long last* (twelve hundred years later) a man was paying her compliments. *And* he looked quite an important man, because people were gathering around and listening to him intently. She had never had so much attention, if she had skin (and all the other bits you need) she would blush!

9.00 p.m.   Watched *Death on the Nile,* starring Peter Ustinov, Bette Davis and David Niven. I imagined Agatha Christie writing her story in Egypt, while she accompanied her my-wife-gets-more-interesting-as-she-gets-older husband, Max Mallowan, on one of his digs.

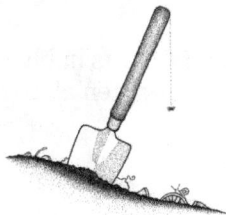

Monday 25th

Ben had the day off work. Autumn sunshine shone on the bonnet of his navy blue Honda Civic (and his bald patch) as he drove off to visit his sister in the beautiful village of Great Tey, near Colchester.

1.30 p.m.   Text message from Ben:

ARRIVED SAFELY AT JULIAS – WILL DO SHOPPIN ON WAY HOME X

2.30 p.m.   With all the excitement of the *double-page spread*, my *witchy website* and watching *Death on the Nile*, I realised I had forgotten to make Ben's birthday card and wrap his gifts.

2.35 p.m.   Started making Ben's birthday card. I thought I'd write the words HAPPY BIRTHDAY, with lettering inspired by the shirts I bought him from Joe Browns catalogue.

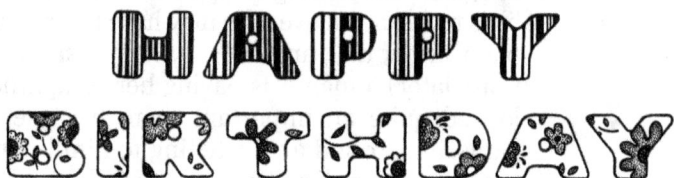

HAPPY BIRTHDAY

The word HAPPY would be colourful. Like the charismatic black Barcelona shirt; with a fun combination of confident-purple, offbeat-blue, charismatic-pink, and totally-self-assured-yellow stripes. The word BIRTHDAY, would be a floral pattern, like the funky floral shirt; a combination of soft greeny-blues, olive greens, purpley-blues and chocolaty-browns.

5.00 p.m.   Wrapped the shirts in blue and silver birthday paper, with BIRTHDAY written all over it, in funky lettering.

BIRTHDAY

6.00 p.m.   Signed the birthday card with Love & Best Witches, from me and the hairy children. Then curled up with my cats for a long doze, relieved I didn't have to prepare or cook dinner.

Tuesday 26th

Ben looked *very cool*, wearing his funky floral birthday shirt today. It really suited him. He said the Barcelona shirt, with the confident-purple, charismatic-pink, offbeat-blue and totally-self-assured-yellow stripes was a bit small. I translated the words 'a bit small' to 'a bit gay'. But this was fine because I had lots of other little birthday treats in mind. I would purchase them at our local garden centre.

Late afternoon, on our way out the front door, I noticed an enormous black house spider with lots of scary legs, sitting sinisterly on the white skirting board by the door. I stayed *very cool*. Closing the front door behind me, I plodded down the path and climbed into the front passenger seat of Ben's car.

As he drove round the corner, out of our street, I mentioned the spider. And at that moment a police car whizzed past with a screaming siren. With all the noise, and the sound of the engine, I misheard Ben's reply.

ME: Did you see that enormously *HUGE* spider near the front door?

BEN: Yeah, I saw him earlier, but I left him a note.

ME: You left him a *NOTE?!*

BEN: No dear, I left him *alone*.

ME: Giggle, giggle. You could have left him a note saying, please vacate the building before we return home.

BEN: *Yeah, hahaha!*

ME: I expect he's at your computer now, making himself at home, checking out websites.

BEN: Or emailing his lascivious lady spider friend, with long legs all the way up to her cephalothorax.

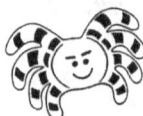

    Ben managed to find a parking space in Notcutts car park, very close to the entrance, which saved a bit of a walk. After wandering through a maze of shrubs, small trees, plants, glazed pots, and garden ornaments with a glazed look in their eyes; we came to the potted-everything section: preserves, chutneys, and pickles. Close by, were the posh crisps, and very mouth-watering fresh cakes. I wanted to purchase *every one*, they looked so delicious, especially the coffee and walnut cake.

ME: Put whatever you fancy in your basket, birthday boy.

BEN: *Great* (eyeing the pretty young sales assistant).

ME: Apart from the sales assistant.

BEN: Yes dear.

    Ben chose ginger conserve, runner bean chutney, spiced garlic pickle, wholegrain mustard, and a fruit cake. I threw a couple of packets of posh snacks into his basket; Stilton and grape chips, and parsnip with black pepper crisps. The drinks section was next to the packets of crisps, so Ben picked up another basket to fill with bottles of Santa's Wobble beer, for Christmas gifts.

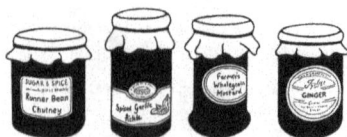

On the way to the checkout, we passed aisles of Christmas goodies: bags of chocolate money, cuddly toys, stocking fillers, festive decorations and festive confectionery. I chose a wind-up penguin and chocolate snowmen, for Louise's Christmas stocking. Then, suddenly, I wanted to lie down on the carpet, curled up with the huge white cuddly toy polar bear, and sleep till Christmas. I've no idea how I got to the checkout counter, and then to our car in the car park. The world went misty, and I felt like I was crawling in a snowstorm, exhausted with hypothermia.

My snowstorm gradually became soft flakes, as we drove through country lanes, past sleepy country cottages and sleepy horses of every horsey-shade, in the fading light. Ben suggested we have a relaxing drink in The Horseshoes pub, where he sometimes does an Avocado Pair gig. He said there's always huge log fires there in the winter, and comfortable chairs. I found the energy to smile and nod in agreement, as I thought about buying a wheelchair. It was about time I treated myself to one. I had recently seen a reasonably priced chrome steel chair, advertised in Healthy Living Direct; it folds up so you can put it in the boot of a car, very convenient. I could float around Notcutts in my heavenly carriage, with a basket on my lap, so Ben wouldn't have to carry our purchases, just push my chair.

ME: I think it's about time I had a wheelchair. I've seen one in Healthy Living Direct, it folds up so you can put it in your car boot.

BEN: Sounds like a good idea.

ME: I've never liked being pushed around by a man, but in this case I'm all for it.

BEN: *Ha ha ha!*

We parked right outside the front door of the pub, which was a relief; much further away, and I'd have had to crawl in like a bumble bee with pollen laden legs. As Ben opened the door, a lovely warm woody smell of wood smoke greeted us. It said, *welcome, come in, take a seat and relax.* I almost fell onto the large squashy sofa, in front of huge inglenook fireplace, with horseshoes nailed onto the beam above a roaring, crackling log fire. While Ben ordered the drinks at the bar, I happily gazed at bright flames licking the logs, and imagined a black cauldron bubbling away.

I moved a cushion from behind my back, and as I sunk more deeply into the sofa, I sleepily surveyed my surroundings, admiring soft lamplight glowing on Stuart tartan upholstery, maidenhair ferns in shiny copper pots, exposed brickwork, and long thin oak beams. Ben admired the maiden serving behind the bar, with shiny red hair, who wore Stuart tartan shorts, exposing her long slim legs. Tarty tartan shorts? At this time of year? Huh.

Jazzy music played quietly in the background, and I hummed along to Sting, singing about an alien in New York. A young couple at a nearby table were glowing with love. Everything seemed to have a golden glow; the drinks on the bar, the logs in the fire, the horse brasses, the mountains of hot chips, piled high on large white plates.

I wondered if The Horseshoes served vegetarian food, most pubs do these days. Though some have just one meal, or a poor selection added on at the end of the menu, like an after-thought to keep the hippies happy. This place was no exception. But I forgave the proprietors, because the pub had such a warm and relaxing atmosphere, with soft seating and lighting, and Sting to serenade me.

The romantic couple, glowing with love and platefuls of hot golden chips, had a large silvery bucket full of ice on their table, cooling their champagne. We had a smaller version of the bucket on our table, full of knives, forks and spoons; like a vase of cutlery flowers. I read the menu again, wondering if Ben would like one of their vegetarian meals for a birthday treat; they looked the sort of olivey-food he likes. There was a choice of rigatoni pasta in marinated artichoke, sun dried tomato, and olive sauce topped with baby basil. Or. Black olive and onion tart, topped with cumin-roasted vegetables, vine roasted tomatoes, crisp home-made onion rings, and smoked tomato dressing.

As Ben headed towards our table with the drinks, I noticed a thin waiter, nervously and profusely apologising to a middle-aged couple two tables away. He looked about twelve, and I felt sorry for him, because the couple looked like Mr and Mrs Most-Miserable. I tried hard to listen to what was going on, my ears were out on stalks because (since I got M.E. with not much of a life) I've become a nosey person. I gleaned from the odd word, that the batter on the seafood was not crispy enough. The waiter said it was something to do with the flour the chef used, although I'm not entirely sure about this. His parting words made me quietly chuckle to myself, but I didn't hear the couple's reply because I was thanking Ben for my drink; a refreshing glass of cold golden cider, to liven me up. I raised my glass to Ben.

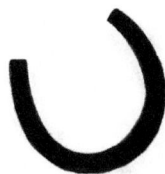

ME: Happy birthday old boy.

BEN: *Cheers!*

ME: *Cheers!* (sip..... sip..... sigh..... smile..... eyes brighten). Look at all the horseshoes on that beam, I like all the different sizes, from Shire to Shetland pony. Isn't the tiny one sweet?

BEN: Yes dear.

ME: We forgot all about that Shire horse fair we were going to go to in the summer. I do love Shire horses, don't you? When I'm admiring a Shire, it's the only time I'm not worried if my bum looks big in my jeans.

BEN: That's nice dear.

ME: Nothing like a *real* log fire.

BEN: You're right there.

ME: The bigger the better, like a Shire horse.

* * * * * * *

We admire the fire, the flames galloping over the logs.

* * * * * * *

ME: A sandwich went into a bar.
The barman says, 'Sorry we don't serve food here.'

BEN: *Ha ha ha!* A man walks into a bar with a roll of tarmac under his arm and says, 'Pint please, and one for the road.'

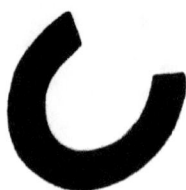

ME: When the man is given his drinks, does he say to the barman, 'Ta, Mac?'

BEN: Very funny dear.

ME: That couple over there, the miserable looking pair, must have complained about their meal. You'll never guess what the waiter said?

BEN: Not in a million years.

ME: He was telling them why the batter wasn't crispy enough, something to do with the flour I think. Anyway, he said the reason *was true*, he got it straight from the horse's mouth. This is The Horseshoes, maybe the chef is a big brown horse.

BEN: What *are* you like.

ME: You see pubs called The Black Horse or The White Horse, you never see The Brown Horse pubs, do you?

BEN: No dear.

ME: Can you look on the internet, to see if there are any pubs called The Brown Horse?

BEN: Yes dear.

ME: A horse goes into a pub and the barman says, 'Why the long face?'

BEN: Is it a brown horse?

ME: In my joke it is...... *sip*...... *sip*...... There's a pub called The Black Horse in the village of Pluckley. I think that's appropriate for a pub in the most haunted village of England.

BEN: The White Horse would be ghostly.

ME: Yes, but in this case it's a black horse that is seen in the pub, it causes objects to vanish and reappear elsewhere. The Coach and Headless Horses would be a good name for a pub in Pluckley.

BEN: Headless horses?

ME: Yes, a phantom coach and horses, driven by a headless man, travels through Pluckley towards Smarden. Some accounts say the horses are headless too.

BEN: Like Headless Nick in the Harry Potter film.

ME: No, he's *Nearly Headless Nick!*

BEN: If you say so dear.... *sip*.... There's a lot of spirits behind the bar here.

ME: I can't disagree with that!

*   *   *   *   *   *   *

We gaze into the flickering flames, casting spooky

shadows on the brickwork.

*   *   *   *   *   *   *

ME: I used to meet up with friends on a Friday night at The Black-smith's Arms. They should have had horseshoes on their beams. I used to call it The Blacksmith's Armpit because the outside toilets were smelly.

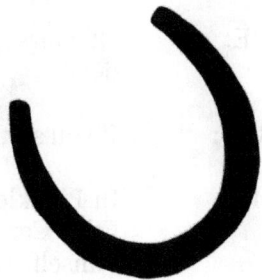

BEN: Maybe the landlord had smelly armpits!

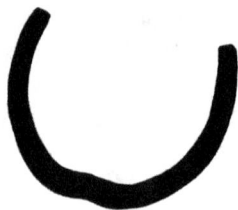

| ME: | He was a rather large sweaty man. His wife had a horsey laugh, and a mane of chestnut hair, that she used to toss when she was angry with her husband. |
| BEN: | Did she gallop about behind the bar? |

* * * * * * *

We laugh as the barman tosses another log on the fire, the flames leaping about, and sparks flying.

* * * * * * *

ME: The horseshoes on that beam are mounted all wrong.

BEN: Why is that?

ME: Well, if they are hung upside down, all your luck falls out, and the other way up, the devil sits in it.

BEN: The devil?

ME: Yes, that's what the Irish say.

BEN: Oh, so that's why the horseshoe above our back door is on its side.

ME: Of course! We will stay lucky and not be tempted by the devil.

BEN: If you say so dear.

ME: In Pluckley, if you dance around the Devil's Bush near Frith Corner, you can make direct contact with Lucifer himself. Dancing around the bush three times evokes a personal appearance, but you have to be completely naked or it won't work. Nobody knows which bush is the Devil's Bush though.

BEN: That's a devil of a shame!

ME: It is for the man who lives in a nearby cottage, is a keen bird watcher, and always has his binoculars at hand, ha ha!

* * * * * *

Feathery flames look hellishly hot, as they dance around the logs.

* * * * * *

ME: This sofa is a nice tartan. I wonder what tartan it is, it's a biscuit colour. They seem to have lots of different tartans in this pub. Can you .....

BEN: Find tartans on the internet, so you can have a browse?

ME: Giggle.... sip.... sip.... Next door had a *most gorgeous* Stewart tartan sofa delivered on Monday.

BEN: Did you covet thy neighbour's sofa?

ME: I most certainly did, the devil would have led me to temptation to order one just the same, but my horseshoe is on its side, so he's unable to sit in it.

* * * * * *

Ben licks his lips as he glances at the menu, I watch fork tongued flames licking the logs.

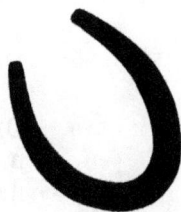

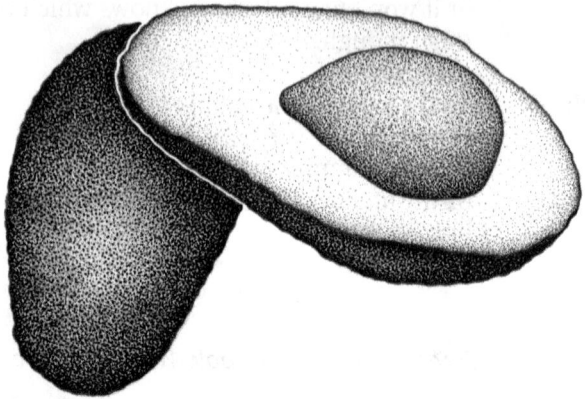

BEN: Jess sent me a good cat quote today: Cats see humans as warm blooded furniture.

ME: Many a true word spoken in jest (big smile).

BEN: Many a true word spoken by Jess.

ME: That's true! Look, there's a picture of a brown horse over the fireplace. If I had a pub I'd call it The Brown Horse. I would have an Avocado night, with the Avocado Pair for entertainment, and all the meals would have avocado in the ingredients.

BEN: Sounds good!

ME: Yes, there would be a choice of avocado and grapefruit salad, avocado stuffed omelette with big fat crispy golden chips, or avocado soup with fresh bread rolls.

BEN: Home-made horseradish sauce, called Horsey sauce?

ME: Of course, and interesting *hors* d'oeuvre; like guacamole made with chillies, onions, tomatoes and avocado, or mozzarella and avocado bees.

BEN: Bees?

ME: Yes, you arrange mozzarella cheese slices between slices of an avocado, to form the striped body of a bee. Then you place semi-circular slices of cheese at the sides, for the wings, and it all sits in a bed of lettuce.

BEN: What about the eyes?

ME: Stuffed olives sliced in half. Oh, and the dressing is olive oil, tarragon vinegar, salt and pepper.

BEN: Sounds marvellous...... You could have a few horseshoe shaped chips to go with it.

ME: Yes! All different sizes, from Shire to Shetland pony..... no need for a side saddle..... I mean side salad..... *giggle*.

BEN: What about pudding?

ME: Hmm....... sip..... sip.... Avocado coloured ice-cream or mousse, served with wafers and lots of little horseshoe shaped plain chocolate pieces.

BEN: Mmm.... sip.... sip.... all different sizes, from Shire to Shetland pony.

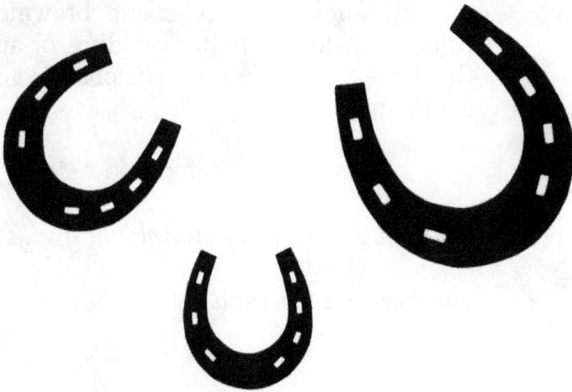

ME: My mum used to put avocado in her custard.

BEN: Are you sure dear?

ME: Ermm..... no..... avocaat..... no..... advocaat!

BEN: I'm feeling hungry now.

ME: Me too. Do you remember the lovely meal we had at The Veggie Red Lion on your fiftieth birthday?

BEN: Yeah, brilliant menu! I had the baked Camembert with horseradish chutney and home-baked bread, as I recall.

ME: Mmm, I remember, and I had the Brie and asparagus cheesecake, followed by the Wellington.

BEN: Wellington? Did you put your foot in it dear?

ME: *Cackle, cackle!* Roasted mushroom Wellington: a whole roasted wild mushroom, stuffed with fresh basil pesto and mozzarella, in a puff pastry. It was served with a lovely white wine sauce. *Heavenly.* What did you have?

BEN: The wild mushroom, port and chestnut pie.

ME: Oh, yes, I remember. And we didn't have any room in our tummies for a chocolate brownie sundae, boozy brioche bread and butter pudding, or apple crumble. All the desserts sounded *so delicious,* I want to go back and eat them all.

* * * * * * *

We enjoy watching the glowing logs crumble, while our tummies rumble.

* * * * * * *

ME: I don't like the name, The Veggie Red Lion, it should be something short, like The Green Salad or The Red Pepper.

BEN: Or Verity Red's Pepper.

ME: Yes!

BEN: The Head Of Lettuce?

ME: Oh, yes, like The Kings Head, but more veggie! It's a cosy pub, maybe...... The Peas In A Pod...... no, that's too long..... The Pea Pod.

BEN: Or Peas In A Pub!

ME: *Giggle..... giggle.....* a pub full of peas..... and carrots..... and onions..... lots of lovely veggie veg..... *giggle..... giggle.*

BEN: The cider bubbles have gone to your head, you've got a bit of colour in your cheeks now.

ME: It's the warmth of the fire too. I do feel better, less of a pale zombie, more like a rosie-cheeked little witch by her fireside, watching nettle soup bubble in her cauldron. Would you like to eat here? Not much of a vege menu, and I'm allergic to olives, but the chips look tasty. I could have lots o'chips!

BEN: *Groan.....* I've got an Avocado gig tonight.

ME: OK, maybe another time. Did you know Lush do a bath ballistic called Avobath, the avocado oil is very moisturising and it's a lovely summery green colour with gold sparkly bits.

BEN: Lovely.

ME: Yes, I may put it on my list for Santa. It's very refreshing, like this cider..... *sip.... sip.....* because it smells of lemon grass, lemons and limes.

BEN: Mmm.

ME: It takes *ten* whole fruits to produce just one teaspoon of avocado pear oil, which is *full* of beneficial fatty acids and vitamins.

BEN: Great.

ME: That extra large shirt is looking tight around your middle, have you been putting too much middle-age-spread on your toast? I *really* must put you on a diet.

BEN: Yes dear.

ME: When you're slimmer you'll have *so much more* energy to do all those little jobs that need doing around the house.

BEN: Of course, anything you say dear.

Me: Wendy of Weekly Wife says eating avocado can help you lose weight.

BEN: Really?!

ME: Yes, I was surprised too. A study from a university in California has found avocado is an ideal choice for dieters, despite the fruit's high fat content. Researchers found that participants who ate half an avocado at lunchtime, felt fuller than those in the control group, so they were less likely to snack between meals.

BEN: *Wonderful*, is it that time? We should head home.

ME: Yes, of course, you need time to *avo* bath before your *avo* gig.

BEN: Lets go then, don't forget your coat.

ME: When I first read that article, I had my M.E. eyeballs in, and you'll never guess what I read.

BEN: Not in a million years dear.

ME: I read that eating a *volcano* can help you lose weight.

BEN: We'll head to one of the Caribbean islands this year then, and I'll get munching. You could help me, you could do with losing some weight too.

ME: Thank you dear.

We *erupt* into laughter.

Wednesday 27th

8.45 a.m.   Woke up feeling exhausted, fatigued and knew *without doubt*, that I would feel worse tomorrow. I would experience the usual relapse, after a trip out of the house, with lots of conversation. Was it worth it? *Yes.*

8.47 a.m.   I knew also, that I wouldn't be able to do much today except daydream and recall my dreams. Last night I wandered through a fairytale garden centre; a maze of pink rose bushes and topiary trees, shaped like jigsaw puzzle pieces. Ben walked beside me, and Alice of Wonderland peered shyly at us from behind a stone statue of the Mad Hatter.

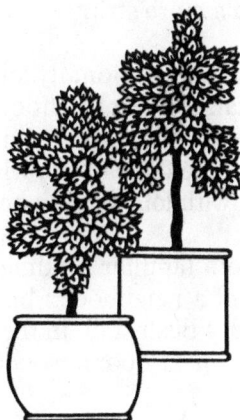

The raspberry-red Cheshire cat sat in a rose bush, grinning widely.

9.14 a.m.   I sipped my morning tea. I crunched my morning toast. I recalled autumn leaves crunching under my feet, as I drifted through the fairytale maze in my dreams. The leaves were silver and shades of blue, the same shades of blue as the flowers on Ben's shirt. I watched in wonder as the blue flowers turned into butterflies, then flew out of his shirt. They settled on the topiary trees, and white statues of Peter Pan, Tinkerbell, Snow White and the Seven Dwarves.

10.05 a.m.   A chilly autumnal wind blew the cat flap open. It was a cold there's-gonna-be-snow-in-November wind. The cat flap has started to make a sad, sort of groaning sound, when it opens wide. A spooky sound. It sent a little shiver down my spine, *most apt* for Halloween. My bare ankles shivered too, but my heart smiled warmly, as I watched a squirrel bounce across the crispy-autumnal-leaf strewn lawn, with a mouthful of peanuts.

10.06 a.m.   I laughed when I noticed her mouth was stuffed so full, cheeks bulging, you could see some of the peanuts. I grinned, as she ferociously dug a small hole in the lawn to bury her collection, grey bushy tail quivering. Then she checked her other small stashes of nutty treasure, dotted here and there, between tufts of grass. She wasn't Nutty, he had a more stripy tail. Maybe I would call her Tufty.

10.07 a.m.   Tufty was occasionally sitting upright, like a miniature meerkat. Her big bright eyes were like shiny black fresh-water cultured pearls, and constantly watchful; well, you couldn't be too careful, with all the huge hairy monsters about, with lots of teeth and claws.

10.08 a.m.   I heard a familiar tinkling sound. It was the bell on the collar of a neighbour's black cat, who wanted to eat the rat with a bushy tail. In the twitch of a whisker, Tufty flew up onto next door's wooden fence. Then she did what I call, playing statues, crouching low and staying completely still.

10.09 a.m.   Then she was away, bouncing along the fence at super squirrel speed. Flying up into the sycamore tree branches, *boing, boing, boing.* I breathed a sigh of relief, as I switched the kettle on, ready for more autumn-watch.

10.10 a.m.   I circled *Autumnwatch* in my TV magazine. Tonight on BBC2, Chris Packham would be revealing how squirrels use deceit and theft to stockpile food for winter. *My* squirrels are good little squirrels, they don't need to use theft and deceit. *My* squirrels have a lovely human to provide for them.

11.45 a.m.   Sam spider sat silently in his website in a corner of the kitchen window. I wondered if he were daydreaming about his lascivious lady spider friend, with gorgeous legs all the way up to her cephalothorax. He solemnly and spiderly watched me open my post.

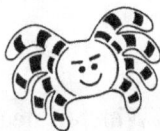

ME: My Halloween stickers should arrive soon. There will be lots of spider pictures, I could decorate your corner.

SAM: Marvellous (spider language).

ME: Are you looking forward to Halloween?

SAM: What are you like (spider language).

12.30 p.m.   Sent a text message to Ben:

B - 2 TIRED 2 COOK 2NITE - CAN U GET FRESH PIZZA ON WAY HOME?

12.34 p.m.   He replied:

                   WILL DO X

1.24 p.m.   Text message from Jayne:

                   HI WITCHY FRIEND, DID U GO OUT 4 BENS B-DAY? WHAT DID U
                   DO?

1.26 p.m.   I replied:

                   HI, YES, WE WENT 2 A GARDEN CENTRE — BOUGHT SUM
                   TREATS AND XMAS GIFTS — HAD DRINK IN COZY COUNTRY
                   PUB — BIG LOG FIRE — VERY TIRED, BUT HAPPY WITCH HUG X

* * * * * * *

7.00 p.m.   Ben sat at his computer.

BEN: There are no pubs called The Brown Horse, but there are
                   two inns, called The Brown Horse Inn.

ME: Really, where?

BEN: One's in Winster, near Lake Windermere, the other is in
                   Brighouse, Nr. Halifax.

ME: We went to The Brown Trout last summer, near the cat
                   holiday home, Lamberhurst way. Do you remember? Nice
                   comfy chairs.

BEN: Yeah.

7.20 p.m.   Ben still at computer.

BEN: Is this the tartan you liked ?

ME: No, too dark.

BEN: What about this?

ME: Almost, could be.

BEN: This? Yes? No?

ME: Not sure, maybe. Very close. Stuart Camel. Hmm, I think I prefer our Stuart Black throw.

BEN: Stuart Black with grey, white and tabby cat hair!

* * * * * * *

7.45 p.m.   Ben lay on the Stuart Black, grey, white and tabby sofa, watching Star Trek.

BEN: If there's an infinite number of stars in the galaxies, and an infinite number of galaxies, in an infinitely large universe, there must be an infinite number of pubs out there.

ME: Of course! *But* there won't be any called The Brown Horse. There may be a Blue Horse or a Little Green Horse, where little green aliens go for a pulsar pint. Did you know, the first pulsar discovered in the sixties, was called L G M, for little green men?

BEN: That's interesting dear.

ME: Yes, Cambridge astronomers likened the radio waves to the kind of signals an alien civilisation might beam into space.

BEN: Marvellous.

ME: In the constellation of Orion, there's a Horsehead nebula, that really does look like a horse's head with a flowing mane.

BEN: So, no doubt, there will be a pub called The Horse's Head somewhere out there.

ME: Yes, and I expect aliens will pop in for a constellation cocktail, and tell jokes about the English, Irish and Scottish astronauts going into a pub.

BEN: Beam me up Scottie!

Thursday 28th

9.30 a.m.   I felt *so* tired, achy and headachy, that I almost crawled to the bird table. A passing woodlouse nearly out-crawled me. I spoke to him.

ME: Hi Woody, I'll be crawling beside you in a moment.

WOODY: What are you like (woodlouse language).

10.05 a.m.   My low spirits lifted a little, like autumn leaves in a November gust of wind, as I watched a squirrel feed on today's new treats. I had put out R.S.P.B. fruity nibbles, because Tesco had run out of peanuts. They were top grade suet pellets, with at least 35% vine fruit. I wasn't sure if the squirrels would approve.
             The doves descended on the bird table first, and appeared to enjoy their fruity snack, as they pecked away *madly*. When a squirrel sprang onto the table they flew away, wings flapping *insanely*. The squirrel wasn't sure about this new food, these pellets were not his usual peanuts. He scratched his little grey head. He picked one up and munched it thoughtfully. He ate another. Then another, munching furiously. He stopped for a squirrelish think, *then* stuffed as many treats into his mouth as he could, and scampered off to bury them on the lawn.

10.30 a.m.   I watched leaves falling from the trees. Two landed on my broomstick. I felt like a sad witch.

             She wandered lonely as a witch

Without her cat, without her broom
Her head a Gothic mansion
Silent, dark, and full of gloom

11.00 a.m. I needed a tasty treat.

11.07 a.m. Sipped de-caf tea in a Kit-Kat mug. Nibbled a finger of Kit-Kat.

11.08 a.m. Nibbled another finger of Kit-Kat. Remembered my foam stickers should arrive any day now.

11.40 a.m. Hurrah!
My foam stickers arrived from Yellow Moon catalogue. The jigsaw-puzzle-shaped alphabet stickers were nice and squidgy and colourful. The Halloween stickers were amusing and very colourful too.

11.43 a.m. I opened the packet of jigsaw puzzle stickers and found: one **B**, two **E**'s, one **H**, one **C**, two **S**'s, one **W**, one **I**, and two **T**'s. I fitted them together, in a higgledy-piggledy-way.

11.44 a.m. I *spelled* out the words, **BEST WITCHES**.

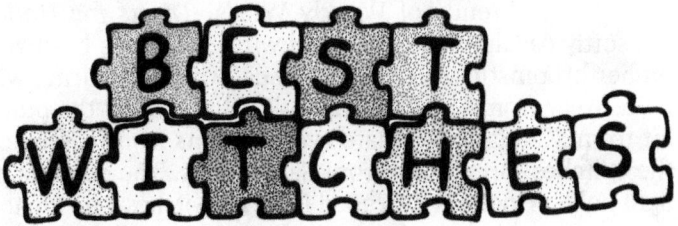

11.48 a.m. Found one **V**, one **E**, one **R**, and one **Y**.

11.52 a.m. Then one **T**, one **I**, one **R**, one **E**, and one **D**. I joined them together to spell out **VERY TIRED**.

12.00 noon. Found more letters and spelt out **VERI TY RED**.

12.02 p.m.   Suddenly I felt *VERY TIRED*.

12.04 p.m.   Snored on the sofa with my cats.

2.14 p.m.   Woke up feeling a little better after witchy dreams. A jig-
               saw puzzle of three witches, riding on their broomsticks,
               came alive. Then the witches flew out of the puzzle towards
               an open window, black smoke streaming from the end of
               their broomsticks. As I watched them fly across a pink and
               golden sunset, the smoke spelt out two words. Best witches.

2.20 p.m.   Mug of tea and playtime with my Halloween stickers.
               Delicious colours: plum-purple bats, lime-green witches,
               juicy-orange pumpkins, apple-green spiders, and creamy-
               white ghosts. The black scaredy cat was my favourite.

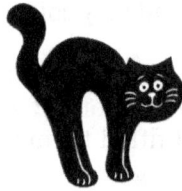

Friday 29th

  Wendy of Weekly Wife's, *Treats for Halloween*, made
me softly cackle; like a tired old witch, who has been riding too long
on her broomstick in October winds, without wearing witchy thermal
underwear from M & S (Magic & Spells). I liked the pumpkin carving
kit from Matalan, chocolate eyeball treats from Tesco, and *especially*
the Witches' Brew soup from Sainsbury's. The ceramic pumpkin tea-
light holders looked like a good idea, for witches who are too worn out to
carve a pumpkin lamp from a real pumpkin. I often make tiny pumpkin
lights, using orange peppers.
  I will ask Ben to see if he can get the New Covent Garden
Witches' Brew soup, from Sainsbury's tomorrow. I'll make creepy
croutons; they will be bat shaped toast, dyed black with food colouring.
The witch in my book makes creepy croutons that are inedible, because
she makes creepy crawlies from burnt toast; but her bat butties are

delicious. They are chip butties with a bat shaped toasted on the top, although her bat shapes are a bit crumby!

I may do a spell using healing oils, candles and herbs (like the witch in my book). I haven't done a spell since last Halloween. Cosmic Colin says this is a *fabulous* time for expressing my *true self.*

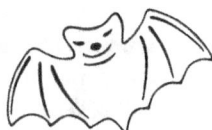

6.14 p.m. Ben printed out an email from Clare at A.F.M.E. who had received my book extracts etc.

Hi Ben,

Thanks very much for this, looks fab! I will let you see a copy of the page proof as soon as we get it.

Best wishes – or rather witches :o)

6.15 p.m. *Ooh, I can't wait!!*

Saturday 30th

Today I was a witch with a big toothy smile, because I am not a toothless old witch. Yet. My morning was brightened by some lovely witchy verse, sent to me by Julia's little granddaughter, Kira.

WITCH

What is a witch?
A witch is a friend
A trusty companion

Ready for secrets and magic to share
So be aware

Verity Writes Again

Cunning and sneaky
A little bit freaky

Potions and cauldrons
Black cats and pointy hats
What's the catch?

Broomsticks and wands
Frogs in ponds
Spiders and webs
Under the bed

It's all here for you to see
So come with me

My witchy world awaits you!!!

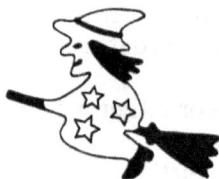

Ben brightened my afternoon, when he arrived home from town with a Sainsbury's bag full of Halloween treats, as well as the usual Saturday shopping. There were sweets for any trick-or-treaters that may call: Cauldron mix, chocolate eyeballs, Cadbury's dead heads, and chocolate pumpkins.

For our Halloween evening, Ben bought plastic goblets; one purple with a spook design, the other green with a bat design. They were beautifully light (for weak, achy hands to pick up) and I wouldn't have to be careful not to break them when I did the washing-up. The orange and black (pumpkin shaped) paper plates, were wonderfully light too, and I wouldn't have to wash them up either!

I was *simply delighted* that Ben managed to get the New Covent Garden Witches' Brew soup, I thought Sainsbury's may have sold out. I read the side of the carton and cackled; the best cackle I had done all year.

WITCHES' BREW SOUP

We've stirred up another smoky storm in our seasonal soup cauldron. We've blended together velvety pumpkin flesh with blood ~ red plum tomatoes; and for a bit of extra bite, cast in a spell of chick peas, kidney beans and black eyed beans (which look just like real eyeballs ~ a great twist for the kid's Halloween parties).

Hubble bubble, fire and ice;
In our cauldron, go all things nice.
No lizard's tongue, or baboon's blood;
Just tasty pumpkins, and the odd spud.
No wing of bat, or eye of toad;
(They're just phrases to help our ode).
In fact, no meat at all; or anything edgy.
Our latest Halloween soup, is suitable for veggies.

We get excited about our themed soups, and Halloween is possibly our favourite occasion. Only great ingredients go into our recipes, but if we really had a cauldron to banish things for eternity, then wasps and slugs (what's the point of either); unpredictable weather; maths exams and frown lines would definitely be on the menu (we're assuming that all the other ills of the world are boiling away, of course).

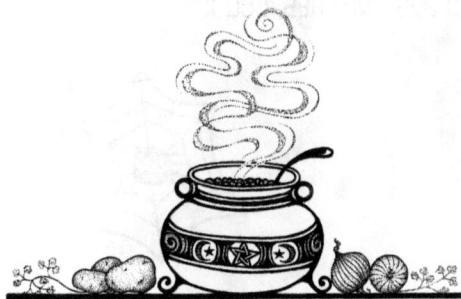

Sunday 31st

8.42 a.m. Text message from Jayne:

HAPPY HALLOWEEN – THANK U SO MUCH FOR YOUR CARD – WILL U BE GETTING UP TO ANY WITCHY SHENANIGANS? HALLOWEEN HUGS XXX

8.43 a.m. I reply:

HAPPY HALLOWEEN – I-M HAVIN WITCHES BREW SOUP WITH CREEPY CROUTONS – CHOC PUMPKINS FOR AFTERS – THEN GONNA WOTCH HARRY POTTER AND THE CHAMBER OF SECRETS – WOT R U DOING?

8.47 a.m. Jayne replied:

WE-RE HAVIN PUMPKIN SOUP AND WOCHIN MY FAVE HARRY P MOVIE – HARRY P AND THE PRISONER OF AZKABAN

8.48 a.m. I reply:

FABULOUS – HAGRID HUGS XXX

11.02 a.m. Text message from my niece:

HAPPY HALLOWEEEEEEEN – LOVE THE CARD, ESPECIALLY THE SPIDER ON THE FRONT HAHA – THE ENVELOPE IS SO NICELY DECORATED I DON-T WANT TO THROW IT AWAY – LOVE AND BEST WITCHES, LOU X

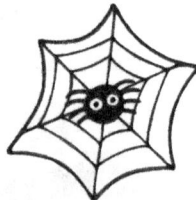

11.04 a.m.   I reply:

> HAPPY HALLOWEEN BEST WITCH, HOPE U HAVE A GR8 TIME
> TRICK-OR-TREATING — WE-RE HAVIN WITCHES BREW SOUP
> WITH CREEPY CROUTONS — LOVE AND BEST WITCHES, AUNTIE
> XXX

11.32 a.m.   Text message from Hannah, Ben's nephew's fiancé. It's her birthday today, and I sent her a copy of my book with her card:

> THANKS FOR THE BOOK AND CARD — BOOK LOOKS VERY NICE
> — LOVING THE PICTURES - I WAS UP EARLY OPENING MY
> PRESENTS — A GOOD DAY AHEAD XXX

11.33 a.m.   I replied, remembering Hannah's dad calls her Pumpkin:

> HAPPY B-DAY 2U, HAPPY B-DAY 2U, HAPPY B-DAY DEAR
> PUMPKIN, HAPPY B-DAY 2U — LOVE AND BEST WITCHES XXX

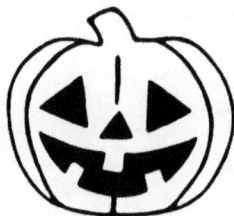

Chapter
Four

November

Hurrah! Ten months! I've survived ten whole months of *another* year; coping with M.E. and myself, *and* trying to care for my man, my cats, and the garden wildlife. Sometimes I wish I *were* having a wild life. But I'm very happy I've managed to keep my sanity for almost another year. Ten out of twelve for me! Soon it will be twelve out of twelve. *Full marks* and a BIG GOLD STAR. A shiny star, like you would find on the top of a Christmas tree.

Christmas. I really can't believe another year is almost over. Soon there will be snow on the ground, Christmas presents to wrap, cards to write, Christmas letters to write, Christmas decorations to put up, Christmas food to buy. I feel exhausted just thinking about it. Fortunately I do all my Christmas gift shopping from home, and I will pace myself with the card and letter writing, present wrapping and festive decorating. When you've had M.E. for years you become an expert at pacing, even if you haven't got the energy to study and become an expert in any other field. I think I could be *very* expert at lying in a field. All.... day...... long................ But not at this time of year, it's getting unbelievably cold. Venturing into the garden is like stepping into a freezer. Brrrrrrrrr.

Today I was snowed under with a flurry of Christmas catalogues, and I merrily fluttered through the pages like a little snow-drop fairy. Do snowdrop fairies flutter through Christmas catalogues? Well, they might. I'm sure my fairies do, because there are a lot of fairy jigsaw puzzles in ACE catalogue: a pink fairy dream castle, pink fairy clock, fairy baking set and Tinkerbell lantern. And *someone* has turned the corner of *those* pages over.

In Yellow Moon catalogue I spotted some new fruit foam stickers, and of course, a creative-card-making-witch always has lots of black card and colourful stickers. And as I always say, the possibilities for creative fun are *simply endless* when you have so much time on your hands. If you have the energy to use your hands, and you can afford foam stickers.

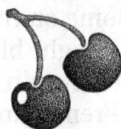

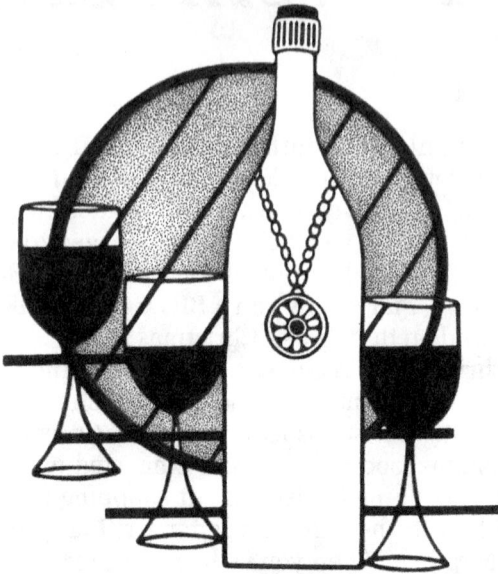

In Scots of Stow catalogue, the authentic looking red wine bottle candle looked like an unusual gift, maybe for one of Ben's family. The wine bottle puzzle was unusual too; not a jigsaw puzzle, but a Woodworkz Wine Puzzle, made from blocks of maple wood. Apparently, fitting the beautiful traditionally made wooden pieces together, and restoring the tactile puzzle to it's bottle shape, will provide a most enjoyable challenge. I'm not so sure about that.

I didn't like the stemless wine glasses either, definitely not a gift I would like to give. They brought to mind rose buds without a stem, and rose buds just don't *look right* without a stem. This is why, when you order roses, you order a number of stems, not buds, because stems are *very* important. I liked the metal wine bottle and glasses wall art though, it would look good in my kitchen.

In Lands End catalogue, I enjoyed *CABLE NEWS: Cardigans now in refined, combed cotton; the texture soft, smooth, and resilient. Shape-keeping, with no trim at cuffs and hems. Effortless to layer.* I imagined wearing the cardie, in nautical blue; sitting on the veranda of my home on the Cornish coast, next door to Dawn French. Wearing the midnight blue cardie, as I watched ships pass in the night on a summer's evening, on my private beach. And I could clearly visualise Dawn French and myself, wearing matching regatta blue cardies as we watched yachts race by, because I had shown Dawn my Lands End catalogue and she had bought four (cardies, not yachts). One in black (because black is slimming) dark grape (to match her favourite wine) pink begonia (for her daughter) and dark sand (for sitting on her sandy beach). I would buy the dark sand cardigan too (for camouflage when I go bird watching on the Cornish coast).

In La Redoute catalogue, the chartreuse green jersey dress with pretty buckle detail, chartreuse satin tunic with appliqué detail, and frilly-front chartreuse top with butterfly sleeves, were lovely. I was *most tempted* to order them all. The chocolate brown, teal green and fuchsia bedspreads, cushions, and curtains, were tempting too.

Instead of reaching for a pen to fill in the order form, I found my Disney jigsaw puzzle, and told myself I felt very inspired, *most tempted*, to piece together the fuchsia bow on Cinderella's fairy godmother's cloak. Also Bashful's teal green hat, Dopey's chartreuse green robe, the chocolate brown part of the Lion King's mane, and Goofy's chartreuse green hat. My Disney puzzle is preventing me from becoming *catalogue-happy*. I will be *puzzle-happy* instead.

7.30 p.m.	*Coronation Street* is exciting; Kevin tells Molly he wants a DNA test, and John gets a shock when he reads a letter in the post.
8.00 p.m.	Ben's news is more exciting — soon there will be a surprise for me in the post.
ME:	Give me a clue, so I've got something to look forward to.
BEN:	No.
ME:	Oh, *please*.
BEN:	It'll spoil the surprise.
ME:	*Pleeeeease* (big sad eyes).
BEN:	No.

ME:	Just a *tiny* clue (bigger sadder eyes, lashes fluttering, head on one side).
BEN:	Oh, *alright*, the surprise will be in an envelope.
ME:	That's not an exciting enough clue.
BEN:	Two tickets.
ME:	Oh goody! Will they be for a band, or one of our favourite comedians.
BEN:	My lips are now sealed.
ME:	As sealed as the envelope with the tickets?
BEN:	Yes, *dear.*

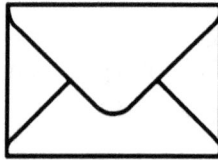

Tuesday 2nd

I wrapped-up warm, to brave the bitterly cold November winds this morning, before feeding the wildlife. Getting wrapped-up didn't mean a hat, scarf, gloves, winter coat and boots. I wore an old jacket with a hood (most useful when you want to hide a bad hair day from the neighbours) over my pyjamas and dressing gown. It wasn't raining, so I wore my slippers. When it rains, I slip on a pair of old shoes. They are like me; flat, worn out, soft, a bit wrinkly, sometimes useful, and they like a little fresh air first thing in the morning, even if it means getting wet.

Back in the comfort of my warm kitchen, with the comfort of my warm cats, I enjoyed a mug of steamy hot de-caf tea, with a steamy hot boiled egg and slice of wholemeal toast. Toast with lots of comforting margarine, making it soggy, like brown autumn leaves in the

rain. My egg was hard boiled because I forgot to time it, my thoughts had drifted away like November clouds, recalling last night's dreams.....
I was sitting at a table in the restaurant where Ben plays, and noticed Tinkerbell jigsaw puzzle pieces floating in my soup.

ME: Waiter, there's a girl in my soup!

WAITER: You ordered the Disney soup madam, it *comes* with puzzle croutons.

The waiter (Peter Sellers) turned into Peter Pan and flew away to the kitchen, where Tinkerbell was tinkling with the cutlery. Then, the waitress (Goldie Hawn) appeared with my queso fritti (breaded brie wedges) that were puzzle shaped.
As I sipped red wine, I noticed the wine bottle and glass artwork on the wall. I gazed transfixed, as the bottle slowly turned and poured chartreuse liqueur into the glasses. Then the glasses drifted away from the wall, to land gently on my table. I smiled, a chartreuse green smile, as the bottle of red wine turned into a candle. I lit the candle, and watched it melt crimson wax all over the crisp white table cloth. I tried to pick up a glass of chartreuse, but it was set firmly in cold crimson candle wax. The stem broke away from my glass, and I was left holding a huge pink rose bud.

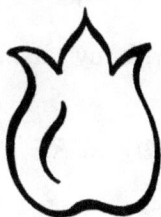

11.00 a.m.   I pieced together strawberry pink roses, in my Disney jigsaw puzzle.

11.00 p.m.   Ben returned home from his gig at the Mexxa Mexxa, with bright pink lipstick on *both* cheeks.

BEN: There were two sweet old ladies, sitting at a table near where we were playing tonight.

ME: Did they wear pink lipstick?

BEN: I don't know, but they must have drunk three bottles of wine between them. They said we were lovely young men, playing our lovely guitars.

ME: That's *lovely*. Did they kiss you on the cheek.

BEN: Yeah, both cheeks.

Wednesday 3rd

9.35 a.m.   In garden feeding wildlife.
             Must remember to put peanuts on shopping list.

9.40 a.m.   In kitchen preparing breakfast.
             Must remember to put peppermint tea on shopping list.

10.10 a.m.   In bathroom brushing teeth.
             Must remember to put Listerine on shopping list.

10.15 a.m.   Sitting on side of bath, resting.
             Will start shopping list in a minute. Peanuts, peppermint, Listerine. Peanuts, peppermint, Listerine.

10.25 a.m.   Lying on sofa with my cats. I have purring in stereo and feel poetic.

             MEEUSIC TO MY EARS

             Purring in stereo
             A sound I love
             The best
             I don't need rock
             Or jazz
             Or blues
             Just pussy cats
             And rest

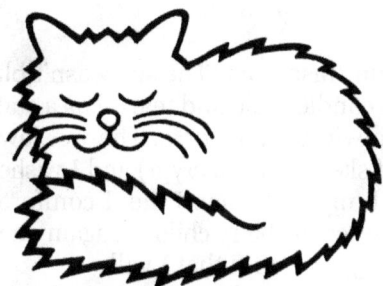

10.36 a.m.	Have forgotten to start writing shopping list. *Peanuts, peppermint, Listerine.* *Peanuts, peppermint, Listerine.*

11.17 a.m.   Postman knocks on the front door with parcel for Ben.

POSTMAN: Good morning, can you sign for this?

ME: Peanuts, peppermint, Listerine.

POSTMAN: Pardon?

Thursday 4th

I waited until the rain stopped drilling into the lawn, to do my usual morning drill. I wrapped-up, then slipped my feet into my flat, old brown shoes, before shivering to the bird table. The weather is as cold as a gravestone on a frosty January morning now.

I found myself standing still, looking down at the two white fairy statues on my cats' graves. The fairies' cheeks were wet. Dark green leaves dripped like the tears of a mourner. My cheeks were dry, but it was raining in my heart, like *the song*. I recalled the lyrics but didn't burst into song, I left that to the birds.

> *The sun is out*
> *The sky is blue*
> *There's not a cloud*
> *To spoil the view*
>
> *But it's raining*

Raining in my heart

The sun wasn't out. The sky wasn't blue. It was pale and solemn as a church candle. Pale and tearful as a statue of an angel in a graveyard, during a winter rainstorm. The wet lawn was strewn with leaves (the colour of skeletons in a crypt) and I wished I could be buried under the lawn with my cats when I die. I comforted myself with the knowledge that I will see my hairy children again one day in spirit, when I pass over — I *know for certain* that I will.

Decided to have fried eggs, mushrooms, tomatoes *and* toast for breakfast (comfort food). And at exactly the same moment as I cracked my egg on the side of the frying pan; the kettle clicked off, the cat flap tapped (as Purrdita padded into the kitchen) and my dragonfly chimes in the garden tinkled. It was a *fun*, almost *musical* moment. My excitement for the day.

10.27 a.m. I admired the Gardener's Cruet Set and watering cans in The Original Gift Company catalogue. They would be an ideal gift for auntie, a perfect accompaniment to the Alan Titchmarsh gardening calendar. They would also match the watering can tea-lights, watering can mobile, and watering can pot holder in my kitchen. I recalled I had admired The Original Gift Company's watering can earrings a few years ago, and shown them to Ben.

10.28 a.m. Remembered our brief conversation.

ME: Aren't these earrings lovely!

BEN: They would pull your ears off dear.

ME: Why?

BEN: They're tablecloth weights.

ME: Oh.

10.46 a.m. I lit a tea-light watering can in my kitchen window. It made me smile. Then I decided to turn the heating up a little; tea-lights make me smile warmly, but they don't give off much heat.

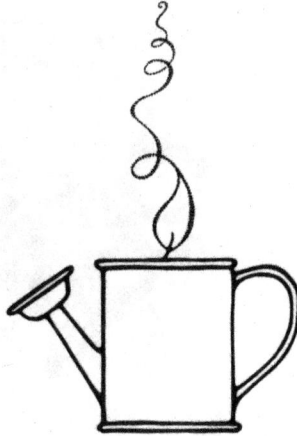

10.48 a.m. I've got a bargain bag of tea-lights, but I can't remember where I've put them. Probably under the stairs somewhere; behind the carpet upholstery cleaner, Bob Martin home flea spray, Mr Sheen, No Nonsense leak sealer, light bulbs, batteries, dinner candles, shoe polish equipment etc.......

10.50 a.m. Wendy of Weekly Wife, told me to warm up my living room with fabulous home buys. I could turn up the heat, without turning up the temperature by mixing rich red, golds, chocolate browns and natural wood.

10.51 a.m. I'll warm myself up instead, with *red* tomato soup for lunch, then I'll have *chocolate brown* chocolate, wrapped in *gold* foil. Good plan.

10.52 a.m. I read that Alan Titchmarsh has a pink and green Sanderson print sofa, with big round arms, and decent cushions that support your head when you are watching TV. Lucky Alan. I wonder if he has a watering can cruet set.

10.54 a.m. Glancing at the fabulous home buys again, I decided the gold candles would look *most fabulous* in my living room, and the wooden clock (with the numbers carved in an arty way) would perfectly match my kitchen cupboards.

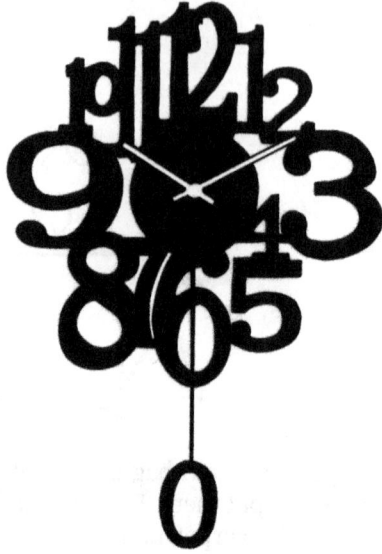

Friday 5ᵗʰ

I was almost blown away by an icy November wind, when I ventured into the garden this morning. A leaf flew onto my cheek, like the slap of an angry spirit's hand. Another landed on my head, light as a snowdrop fairy landing on her feet. Then one more, like the comforting touch of a winter angel, rested lightly on my shoulder. Was this a good sign? I decided it was.

Late afternoon, I watched the *Alan Titchmarsh Show* with guest actress Phyllida Law. When the Saturdays appeared to sing, I switched channels to watch *Loose Women*; Dawn French was a guest, talking about her new book. She said she writes long hand, like me. There are still some of us left. I will put her book on my list for Santa, it sounds *really good* and I *know* it will make me cackle. A lot.

It was a noisy evening. Firework night. This made it difficult to concentrate on *Coronation Street*, because of all the banging and crackling, and sounds like angry ghosts being evicted from their Gothic mansions. But I still enjoyed Sophie's party getting out of hand, and Kevin handing over the DNA test results to Molly.

Mary and Purrdita hid behind sitting room chairs, like my little brother used to, when the Cybermen appeared on *Dr Who*. I must admit, sometimes I feel like hiding behind the sofa when Ben is watching *Dr Who*. Cleopatra wasn't bothered at all by the firework displays, now that she has a wonderful warm and safe home.

7.45 p.m.   I remembered a joke.

ME: Police arrested two kids yesterday.

BEN: Did they dear.

ME: Yes, one was drinking battery acid, and the other was eating fireworks. They charged one and let the other one off.

Saturday 6th

Dawn French was smiling brightly on the cover of my new Weekly Wife. I read the article entitled: *Why Dawn is smiling again!* She is back in the dating game, now that her divorce from Lenny Henry is final. I'm sad that Dawn is divorced after twenty five years of marriage, but their split was amicable and they are still friends, so I'm not *too* sad. She will soon be teaming up with Jennifer Saunders to do a show on Radio 2, to be broadcast on Boxing Day, New Year's Day, and 3rd January. A *must-listen*. Her first novel is entitled: *A Tiny Bit Marvellous*. I think it will be a huge lump of marvellousness, and that's nothing to do with her size twenty frame.

Read tonight's programmes in today's TV Quick magazine. The team on *Coast* will be exploring the Inner and Outer Hebrides, and Kate Row will examine the bone-eating snot-flower worm. A *must-watch*.

In Healthy Living Direct catalogue, I saw a few *must-buys*, and made a list:

1.   Men's thermal socks, for Dad and brother.

2.   No-frost windscreen cloth (specially treated to help prevent frost formulation) for Ben and Dad.

3.   An emergency blanket that reduces risk of hypothermia. For Ben and Dad, in case they are stranded miles from home in the snow, or need to save someone else's life. I have a feeling it's going to be a harsh winter.

Sunday 7th

          The proof copy of my double-page spread arrived today, in the form of a jigsaw puzzle. Dawn French and Jennifer Saunders helped me piece it together as we sat around a fire, dressed as three witches with pointy hats. We all cackled when the puzzle was completed. Then I awoke, wondering when the proof copy would arrive from A.F.M.E. I had a feeling that (like the snow) it would be very soon.
          As I signed two copies of *Love & Best Witches* for Dad and auntie (ready to parcel-up) I remembered there were some amusing quotes about books and writers in my book of quotations.

3.00 p.m.   Find book of quotations.

3.03 p.m.   Find favourite quotes about books and quietly cackled to myself.

          Outside a dog, a book is a man's best friend. Inside a dog it's too dark to read.

          GROUCHO MARX

          A classic is something that everybody wants to have read but nobody wants to read.

          MARK TWAIN

          On the day when a young writer corrects his first proof sheets, he is as proud as a schoolboy who has just got his first dose of pox.

          CHARLES BAUDELAIRE

3.10 p.m.   I recall reading some of Charles Baudelaire's poetry when I was a teenager. It was so beautiful, I decided I could *really* fall in love with a man bestowed with such a gift. I wondered if he did book signings, I *longed* to meet him. I could imagine him asking my name (with a softly sensual and fabulously French accent) before he signed my copy of his latest book of poetry. As our eyes met, I would quote some of his verse (in my best husky voice) and there, in the middle of Waterstones, Charles and I would fall hopelessly in love.

Wearing Maybelline's *Fard à joues lumière* on my cheeks, and *beige rosé* on my lips, I would smile brightly. Then he would tell me that my smile was dazzling, like springtime sunshine on a fast flowing stream. And my eyes were a greeny-blue, like the ocean on a summers day; surrounded by a darker blue, like the distant horizon where the ocean meets the sky.

He once wrote in one of his poems, that he wanted his gaze to *dive into the cold live pools of a cat's enchanted eyes*. When he gazed romantically into my eyes, he would want to dive into their calm and tranquil seas. Then maybe swim to their deep blue horizons, and fall over the edge of the world in love — or something like that. I was most disappointed to discover he had died over a hundred years ago. Hmm, just my luck.

3.15 p.m. I put the kettle on for a de-caf coffee, wishing I were sitting outside a French café in Paris, drinking in the atmosphere with my café latte.

3.20 p.m. I'm browsing through La Redoute catalogue, and find myself thinking of my beloved Charles again. He would have adored me wearing feminine La Redoute fashions. A flowery rose print skirt, candy-floss-pink camisole, floaty sea-green Marianne James dress, or flirty *Jolie Parisienne* deep-purple French knickers.

4.10 p.m. I notice the Eiffel Tower wall art in The Original Gift Company catalogue. It would look *magnifique* next to my Chat Noir café poster, or my oil-on-canvas painting of a French café.

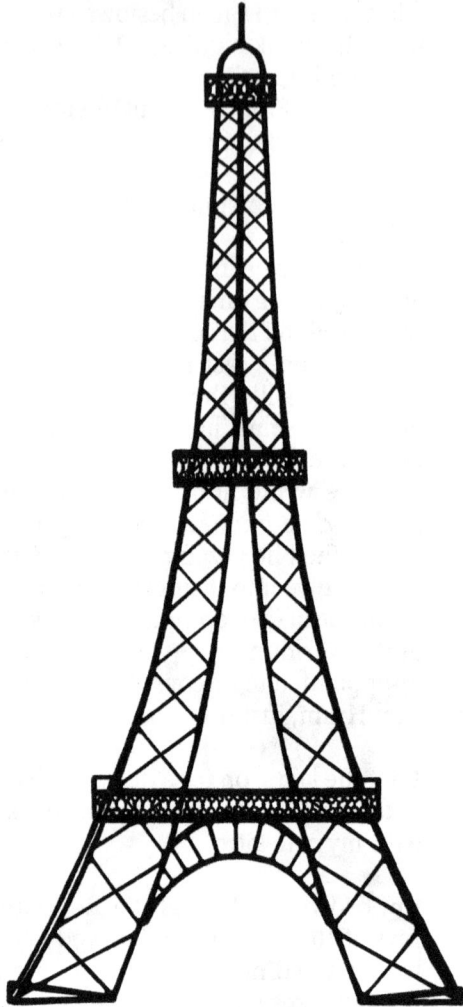

4.11 p.m.   Charles would have proposed to me on top of the Eiffel Tower. I would have smiled and said, 'Oui', my sea-blue eyes shining with *larmes de joie*.

4.12 p.m.   On top of the tower, I would feel on top of the world (as if I were floating on a pearly-white cloud) with my Marianne James dress fluttering in a womanly-warm French breeze.

The sun would come out from behind the clouds at that moment, and sparkle on my engagement ring; a huge heart-shaped cluster of sapphires and aquamarine crystals, surrounded by diamonds.

I would recite some verse that I had written only days before, because I knew *(just knew with all my heart)* that my dearest Charles would propose to me very soon, and he would recite a poem he had written about a cat, because he knew it was my favourite. And after we married, we would live *happily ever after* in Paris with lots of cats, naming our first three after the cats in the film, *Aristocats*. There would be French posters on our walls, like the ones the witch has on her walls, in *Love & Best Witches*. The cats in her posters blink their eyes when there's magic in the air. Our posters would be full of blinking cats every day, because there would *always* be magic in the air when we were together.

Come, lovely cat, and rest upon my heart
And let my gaze dive in the cold
Live pools of thine enchanted eyes that dart
Metallic rays of green and gold

CHARLES BAUDELAIRE

Monday 8th

Pamphlets fluttered through the letterbox today, like colourful rectangular autumn leaves, telling me to stock up for Christmas. Cleopatra flew in through the cat flap, with a sycamore leaf stuck to the fur of her (now) well rounded tummy. I sat contemplating my well rounded tummy, looking forward to Christmas cards flying through the letterbox, and Christmas treats making my tummy more well rounded. I couldn't look forward to *Coronation Street*, because Jack Duckworth was going to die in tonight's episode. I felt so sad, I had to tell Ben when he came home from work.

ME: I can't watch *Coro* tonight.

BEN: Why's that?

ME: Jack's going to die.

BEN: I remember when Vera died, the girls at work were upset.

ME: *Coro* lovers wept all over the country.

BEN: There will be more tears tonight.

ME: Yes. Sniff, sniff. *Coro* won't be the same without Jack and Vera.

BEN: What will you watch instead, to ease your grief dear?

ME: *Ghost hunting* with Yvette Fielding. She's visiting spooky locations in Wales; a clock tower and a manor house.

BEN: You'll get really scared and have nightmares.

ME: I know, and it will serve me right!

BEN: *Yeah.*

ME: The Queen watches *Coronation Street*, I wonder if she'll be a little tearful tonight.

BEN: Probably sniffing into her crisp royal hankie, embroidered in one corner with *H.R.H.*

ME: She likes to have supper on a tray while watching TV. I wonder if she eats when *Coro* is on. Mmm, I think our Queenie may be too upset to have much of an appetite tonight. Although she may have a milky drink later, using her favourite 1953 Royal Coronation cup and saucer, or *Coronation Street* mug (celebrating fifty years of the programme).

BEN: And a Hobnob biscuit.

ME: Or a plain *Rich* Tea. I know she likes plain meals, so that could be a favourite.

BEN: Yes dear (Basil Fawlty voice).

ME: I saw a photo of her a few years ago, on the set of *East Enders*, outside the Queen Victoria pub with Barbara Windsor. I wonder if our Queenie is an *Enders* fan too.

BEN: What are you like.

Tuesday 9th

After a night of nightmares, ghost hunting with Barbara Windsor and the Queen, I read my stars. Cosmic Colin informed me that I had some momentous decisions to make. He was *so right*.

9.20 a.m.   Shall I wear my back-to-school navy blue hair scrunchie, or the bottle green one. I have red and orange scrunchies now, they are energy giving colours. Maybe I'll wear one of them!

9.21 a.m.   The red or orange scrunchie?

9.30 a.m.   Red or orange peppers on tonight's pizza?
Maybe both, that will be exciting.

9.31 a.m.   We have a green pepper too. I'll use all three colours, for a traffic lights pizza.

9.35 a.m.   I'm sitting in the kitchen, gazing at red, green and orange peppers on the work surface, admiring their vibrant colours and sensual shape. Later I will enjoy their fresh peppery aroma, when I slice them up. They taste *so perfect* on a pizza.

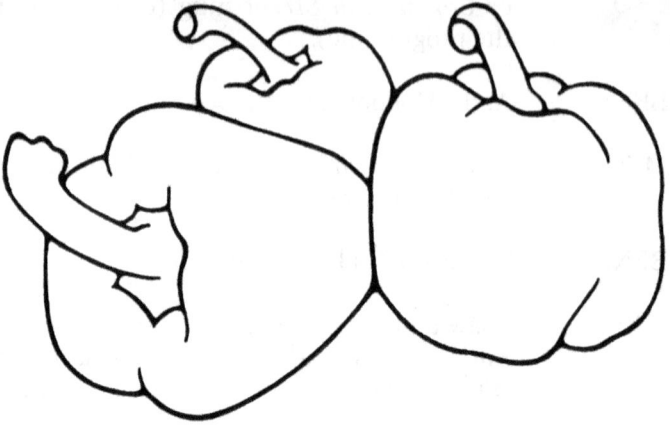

9.36 a.m.   Ben thinks pepper stalks look a bit phallic. I'm a good girl (brought up as a Christian) so of course that thought didn't occur to me at all. I won't tell Ben that the shape of the green pepper brings to mind his bum.

9.37 a.m.   Still sitting, recalling the fun I've had cooking with peppers. If you slice a red pepper in a certain way, you can create nice heart shapes that look effective with a Valentine's Day meal. Ben is always *most* delighted.
             If you slice the bottom off a green pepper, it looks a little like a four leaf clover — just right for a wishing-you-luck meal.

9.39 a.m.   Standing at the kitchen sink, smiling at my broomstick leaning against the garden fence, and my old cauldron that has weeds growing in it now.
             Since I became ill with M.E., making pumpkin lanterns is too exhausting; but it's just as much fun to cut the eyes, nose and mouth out of an orange pepper for Halloween. Although if you are a sensitive witch, this might make you feel sad for a moment; because when you cut the eyes out, the juice looks like tears. When you cut the nose out, the juice looks like the pumpkin face has a cold. And of course, the mouth looks like it's dribbling.

9.41 a.m.	Still standing at the kitchen sink watching the squirrels leaping around in the tree branches, like little hairy gymnasts. When we host the Olympics in 2012, I'll slice different coloured peppers and arrange them on a pizza — five circles, Olympic style. Ben will be absolutely *thrilled*.
9.50 a.m.	Maybe I'll wear a red, orange *and* green scrunchie tonight, for a traffic lights pony tail. I need to lighten-up sometimes.
10.00 a.m.	Shall I use kitchen roll with the brown, orange and red autumn leaf pattern. Or the funky green fish design. I'll go wild and *use both!*
11.10 a.m.	Peppermint or de-caf tea? I'll drink Ben's coffee. It's not de-caf, so I'll be a little wild and hyper-active. Well, as hyper-active as you can be when you have M.E.
11.45 a.m.	In bath.
11.46 a.m.	Shall I use my Sea Vegetable soap (with lime and lavender to balance the ebb and flow of my mind) the seaweed softening my skin. Or the Bohemian soap (for artists and writers) a refreshing lemon soap for clarity of mind?
11.47 a.m.	I will use the Bohemian soap, so I can be wild with clarity, and hyper-actively chop up colourful peppers to sprinkle creatively all over a giant pizza.

Nothing is more difficult, and therefore more precious, than to be able to decide.

NAPOLEON BONAPARTE

6.15 p.m.

BEN: Something smells nice.

ME: That's the traffic lights pizza.

BEN: What will you think of next dear.

ME: There are multiple traffic lights on this packet of spicy houmous and crunchy veg wraps, with Moroccan style chutney.

BEN: Of course there are dear.

ME: Here, look. The red circle with an exclamation mark is allergy advice. The green circle with a **V**, means suitable for vegetarians. And the amber speech bubble has, TRY ME! written inside, with a note saying they're *sure* we'll love the product. If we don't, we can simply return it for a full refund.

BEN: Well, that *is* wonderful news dear.

ME: Yes, but I wouldn't want to be the person in the complaints department receiving half eaten, smelly congealed food. I wonder if anyone sends just crumbs with the wrapper, and a letter of complaint.

BEN: Probably.

ME: I wonder if anyone says in their letter that the Moroccan style chutney is not Moroccan enough. Not enough chillies, coriander or ginger. Or too much grated carrot, spoils the delicate flavour of the yoghurt and mint mayonnaise. Or there's insufficient houmous. And they get a letter back saying, they will not be receiving a full refund because they had eaten all the product, so they must have enjoyed it.

BEN: You have far too much time to ponder.

6.20 p.m.

ME: You know that Phood phone mains charger you ordered for me?

BEN: Mm.

ME   It has ingredients written on the back of the box.

BEN: I'm sure it has dear.

ME: It has! Under the heading, ingredients, it says that the charger is not for human consumption, and why not try other tasty *Phoods*. They do batteries, car chargers, and they have more tasty varieties coming soon. I like their sense of *houmous*. And there's funny little drawings too.

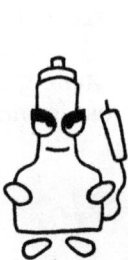 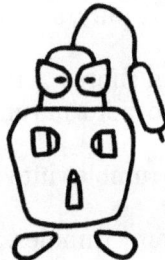 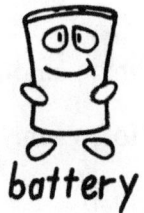

car charger   battery

BEN: Very amusing dear.

ME: Do you like my traffic lights hair style?

BEN: Very nice dear, very, er... colourful.

ME: I've been thinking; on the long road to recovery from illness, you come across many traffic lights and often have to just stop, whether you like it or not.

BEN: What *are* you like.

Wednesday 10th

8.45 a.m.   We've run out of toothpaste.

8.46 a.m.   Find a new tube of Pronamel toothpaste in bathroom cabinet — the toothpaste that protects against enamel erosion. There's a set of traffic lights on the side of the box. A red triangle with a glass (wine acid), a yellow triangle with a lemon (fruit acid), and a blue triangle with a can (acidic drinks). Fabulous. I will point this out to Ben when he comes home from work. He will be *most enamelled.*

10.00 a.m.   Lying on sofa, dozing to the distant sound of the washing machine rumbling in kitchen land.

10.10 a.m.   Lying on sofa, delighting in the sound of Purrdita's soft rumbling purr, as she drifts of to cat dreamland.

10.20 a.m.   Purrdita snores. I lie awake, listening to the sound of a November storm rumbling across farmland.

10.30 a.m.   A lorry rumbles into town.

10.40 a.m.   My tummy rumbles.

10.41 a.m.   Shall I write some verse about the sound of rumbling?

10.42 a.m.   No. I'll have a biscuit. Instead of pouring my heart onto paper, I will pour a cuppa and sit watching the pouring rain.

10.43 a.m.   Shall I write some verse about the sound of purring and pouring?

10.44 a.m.   Or purring and snoring?

10.45 a.m.   No. Not today.

11.30 a.m.   HURRAH!

I text Ben:

THE TICKETS HAV ARRIVED – I-M REALLY EXCITED –
THANX X

12.34 p.m. Ben replies:

GREAT – I-M LOOKING 4WARD TO THE SHOW TOO X
6.10 p.m.

ME: Can't wait to see Bill Bailey, best comedy act *ever*.

BEN: Yeah!

ME: I'll try to rest as much as poss, so I'll have the energy to get to the theatre *and* enjoy the show.

BEN: Good idea.

ME: Yes.

BEN: This will make you laugh. Two cannibals were eating a comedian. One turned to the other and said, 'Does this taste funny to you?'

ME: *Cackle, cackle!*

Thursday 11th

9.40 a.m. The wind was so strong, I almost fell over when I ventured into the garden.

11.00 a.m. The eleventh hour, of the eleventh day, of the eleventh month. I touched the red paper poppy with a black middle, on the mantelshelf. And remembered. I remembered my war veteran friend and his sad stories.

*Kites rise highest
against the wind, not with it.*

WINSTON CHURCHILL

*I went to my doctor
and asked him for
something for persistent
wind. He gave me a kite.*

LES DAWSON

3.00 p.m.   I admired the blowing tree metal wall art in ACE catalogue. A modern tree design with multi-tonal leaves.

3.14 p.m.   Noticed the lawn was now completely covered with leaves.

3.15 p.m.   I imagined the blowing tree wall art in my living room, one leaf dropping off every day. That would be fun.

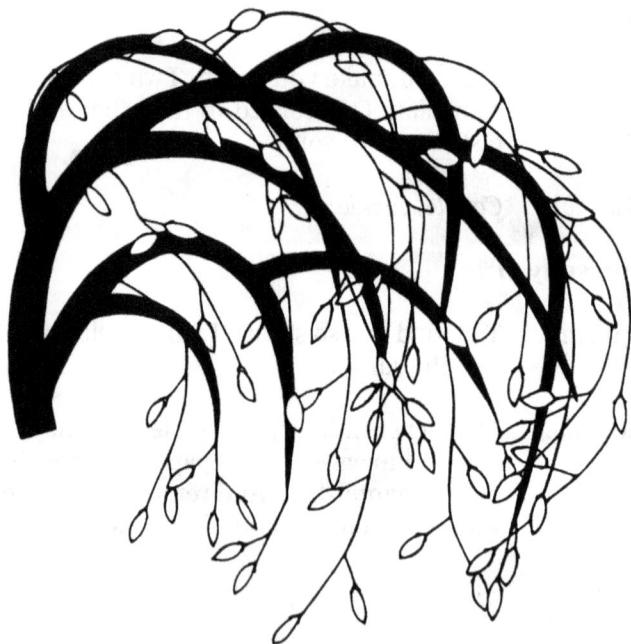

Friday 12th

6.10 p.m.   Oooh, hurrah! *Hurrah! Hurrah!! HURAHHHHHH!!!!!!*

6.11 p.m.   Wonderful! *Wonderful!!! WITCHILY WONDERFUL!!!!*

The proof copy of my double-page spread arrived from Clare at A.F.M.E. Ben printed out the email for me when he got home. Clare asked what we thought, and thanked us for the copies of *Love & Best Witches* we sent for the reader give-away.

ME: It looks great doesn't it!

BEN: Yeah! I like the bats flying round the text.

ME: *Cackle, cackle!* And the photo of the witch with her spell books, candles and potions looks really good.

BEN: Goes well with the photo of you in your witchy hat.

ME: Yes it does! Can you reply to Clare soon as poss, telling her how thrilled I am with my *double-page spread*.

BEN: Will do!

Saturday 13th

2.10 p.m.   Received a text from Jayne:

> HEY WITCHY FRIEND – IF I TOLD U ABOUT THE STUPID STUFF I-VE BEEN DOING, U-D GET ON UR BROOMSTICK – FLY OVER TO KICK MY BUTT WITH UR POINTY WITCHY SHOES – SO TO SAVE U THE WORRY – THE TRIP – LET ME JUST SAY I-VE BEEN OVER ESTIMATING HOW MUCH I CAN DO, BUT HAV HAD A REALITY CHECK SO WONT BE DOING THAT AGAIN IN A HURRY – HAD A PEEK AT UR WEB SITE – IT LOOKS FABULOUS – IT IS VERY U – I MADE IT THRU 3 – 45 OF UR BOOK BUT WAS THEN TOO

ILL TO READ - I SAW THE POSTER FOR THE NEW HARRY POTTER MOVIE - MADE ME THINK OF U - HAGRID HUGS X

2.14 p.m.   I reply:

HI NAUGHTY WITCH, YOR TEXT MADE ME CACKLE - I HOPE U WILL RECOVER VERY SOON FROM OVERDOING IT - I-M GONNA PROBLI OVERDO IT NXT WED - GOING 2 COMEDY SHOW IN LONDON - SO GLAD U LIKE MY WITCHY WEB-SITE - HOPE 2 HAV MUSIC ON IT AND A LINK 2 YOR WITCHY SITE THIS WEEKEND - MY DOUBLE-PAGE SPREAD LOOKS FAB - HAPPY WITCH HUG X

A true friend is one who
likes you despite your achievements.

ARNOLD BENNETT

Sunday 14th

1.45 p.m.   Received text from Ben's sister:

HI - I-VE PUT KIRA-S REVIEW ON AMAZON VIA MY NEW ACCOUNT - LOVE J XXX

1.46 p.m.   I reply:

OH, THAT-S LOVELY - THANX SO MUCH JULIA - THANX TO LITTLE KIRA TOO - LOVE AND BEST WITCHES X V X

2.05 p.m.   I just *have* to text Julia again:

HI, BEN HAS JUST SHOWN ME KIRA-S REVIEW ON AMAZON - IT-S BRILLIANT - I-LL WRITE AND THANK HER ON MY SPECIAL WITCHY PAPER TODAY - BEST SMILING WITCHES X V X

3.45 p.m.   Received a text from Ben:

November

I-M IN SAINS-B – DO U FANCY A CELEBRATION TREAT?

3.01 p.m.   OOH, YES – BUBBLY, THANX X

Come quickly,
I'm tasting the stars!

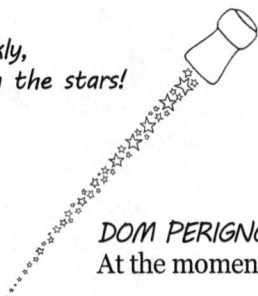

DOM PERIGNON
At the moment he invented champagne.

Monday 15th

10.00 a.m.   I sat watching a centipede crawling across the kitchen floor, on its way towards the back door.

10.01 a.m.   Purrdita padded into the kitchen watching the progress of the tiny creature, so I picked it up carefully. The tiny legs tickled the palm of my hand, then it stopped to listen when I spoke.

ME: You must spend a fortune on shoes, I hope you haven't got designer taste.

CENTIPEDE: Silly human, don't you know there's a discount store in fairyland at the bottom of your garden, called Mataland. The more feet you have, the bigger the discount (centipede language).

11.28 a.m.   Boring post today, lots of brown and white envelopes. More paperwork.

2.17 p.m.   Interesting parcels arrive. A Christmas gift for my niece and newly married friend — a jumper with red hearts, and rainbow coloured LOVE wall art.

LOVE

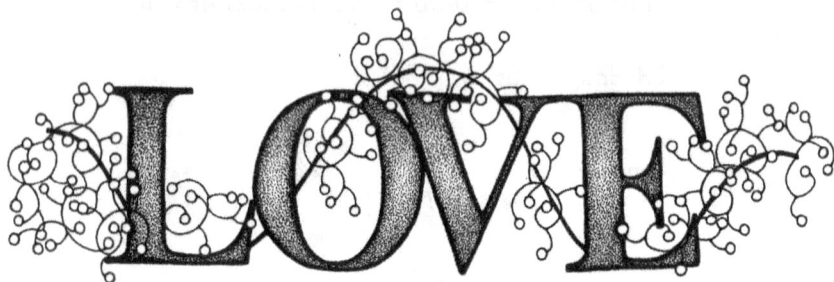

*What the world really needs
is more love and less paperwork.*

PEARL BAILEY

Tuesday 16th

I felt quite good today, but resisted the urge to overdo-it, cleaning the cooker and bathroom sink. I need to stock up as much energy as possible for my trip to see Bill Bailey; about an hours journey, and I'll lie down on the back seat of our car while Ben drives. Luxury.

11.00 a.m. Sitting in kitchen. Watching squirrels dancing and swinging through the trees, and ignoring the cooker that looks like it hasn't been cleaned since the swinging sixties.

11.03 a.m. I will find the fruit foam stickers from Yellow Moon catalogue, and have fun sticking them on the fridge door.

11.23 a.m. Have found the stickers. Sipping strawberry and mango tea for inspiration.

11.24 a.m. I like the strawberry, pineapple, grapes and cherries best. The bright red, yellow, green and purples, will look good on the white fridge door.

11.25 a.m. The fridge door is not as white as it should be.

11.26 a.m. Resisting urge to clean fridge door. And inside of fridge.

11.30 a.m. I think I'll decorate our old Tupperware boxes. The apple, pear, orange and banana will look good on the faded blue lids.

11.38 a.m. I smile. A job *well done.*

11.40 a.m. Resisting urge to clean out cupboard where the Tupperware boxes are kept.

11.45 a.m. Sitting, watching the collared doves feed, I'm resting peacefully from my morning's excitement.

11.50 a.m. My black witchy saucepans would look good with red and yellow fruit stickers (well, until the heat melted them).

11.52 a.m. Just noticed there's raspberries, blackberries, and kiwi fruit slices in the sticker packet. I must use them.

11.55 a.m. I'm tempted to decorate the odd cupboard, white cooker and washing machine. No. It's not a good idea to get *too* fruity in the kitchen; unless you are Glenn Close, and starring in the film, *Fatal Attraction.*

1.30 p.m. Sitting in the kitchen again. Sipping peach and passion fruit tea, and wondering if you can buy vegetable foam stickers from Yellow Moon catalogue, the old vegetable rack could do with cheering up.

1.34 p.m. Feeling inspired. We have a white fruit bowl somewhere. It's quite large, I could use *all* the fruit stickers. Good idea. But I think I'll save that fun for another day.

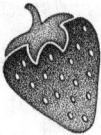

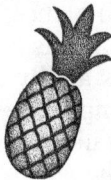

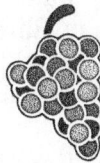

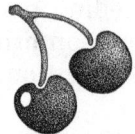

2.00 p.m.   I curl up with my cats, and this week's copy of Weekly Wife. The actress Tamzin Outhwaite grins out of the double-page spread (not *half* as good as *my* double-page spread). She is working with PinkRibbonBingo.com, to raise money for Breakthrough Breast Cancer, and has a full body check at the doctors every three years. I must make an appointment for a breast cancer check, when I've recovered from my trip to London.

Never go to a doctor
whose plants have died.

ERMA BOMBECK

    Tamzin has just completed a successful run in London's West End musical, *Sweet Charity*. I will be in London's West End tomorrow. *Hurrah, can't wait!*

Wednesday 17th

    Cosmic Colin told me to be adventurous, the trip would be worthwhile. He was *so right.* I had the *most wonderful* evening at the theatre, despite the tiring journey (the rumbling on the motorway made me feel ill).
    When we arrived in London, it didn't take too long to find a parking space in the multi-storey car park, but the flight of stairs out of the car park, were a *different* story. Five gruelling flights of eight steps. I had to keep sitting halfway up the stairs for a rest, I couldn't take the lift. I avoid lifts since I got trapped in one, but that's *another* story.
    At one point, I think it was during the third flight of steps; I sat down with my head in my hands, and said a *very naughty* word, with frustration at my lack of energy. Then I had the distinct *horrible* feeling I was being watched, and glanced up to see a camera on the ceiling, pointed in my direction. I was *so embarrassed*, the security person probably thought I was a silly drunk female. Drunk with exhaustion, yes. Drunk with champagne — sadly, no.
    It was a freezing walk to the theatre, but luckily I had wrapped-up well, and wore my flat woolly boots. It started to sprinkle with rain as we emerged from the car park (and I had forgotten my

umbrella) so my woolly boots would have become soggy boots, but fortunately the walk was short and (*even more* fortunate) the theatre was below ground level, with only two little staircases going down.

The venue was small, warm and dark. Really cosy. Lovely. And it felt good to settle into a comfortable seat near the stage, not (what seemed like) miles away, when we saw Bill perform in Brighton.

Although the show was brilliantly entertaining, sitting upright quickly became unbelievably tiring. I wanted to lie down on the carpet by the bar during the interval. *Again,* a security person would think I was drunk. Drunk with embarrassment, yes. Drunk with the finest Scottish whiskey — sadly, no.

Ben bought me half a pint of cider during the interval, he was my knight with a shiny glass. The sparkling, golden and refreshing drink, gave me the energy to stay vertical and keep my eyes open. Also to clap. Well, a sort of clap. When I go to the theatre, I touch the palms of my hands together when the audience claps, because clapping is exhausting and makes my fatigue worse. More importantly, I don't want the stranger sitting next to me to think I can't be bothered to show my appreciation. I think my constant cackling showed a lot of appreciation though; I can't remember when I last laughed so much, with tears streaming down my witchy face. Yes I can. It was the last time I saw Bill Bailey in concert.

After the show, I left the theatre in a sleepy up-lifted haze; then dozed all the way home, recalling the funniest parts of the evening and giggling to myself. We arrived home safe and sound, close to midnight. I was ready to crawl slowly up to bed, like a sleepy snail. Ben was ready for a midnight snack, like a hungry wolf.

Midnight.

ME: Bill always makes me cry with laughter, I'm glad I brought a big supply of tissues.

BEN: Mm. Munch, munch.

ME: Laughter with tears (like sunshine on a rainy day) creates a rainbow of happiness.

BEN: Yes dear.......*y*.....*a*.....*w*.....*n*

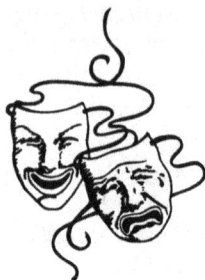

Thursday 18th

8.25 a.m.   Feeling like a zombie, I somehow managed to feed the wildlife and my cats. Too exhausted to feed myself, I plodded, then half crawled back upstairs to bed.

1.00 p.m.   Received a text from Jayne:

        HI WITCHY FRIEND, HOW WAS UR SHOW?
        WOT DID U GO SEE?

1.03 p.m.   I replied:

        SHOW WOZ FABULOUS – WENT TO SEE BILL BAILEY COMEDY
        ACT – CACKLED A LOT – IN BED RECOVERING NOW – TIRED
        HAPPY WITCH HUGS X X X

1.10 p.m.   I texted Ben:

        2 TIRED 2 COOK 2NITE – CAN U GET SUMTHIN ON WAY
        HOME PLZ?

1.21 p.m.   WILL DO X

1.22 p.m.   THANX X

November

2.00 p.m.   Oh God. *Oh God! Oh God! Oh God!* I am *so bored.* B....
O.... R.... E.... D. But *more* bored than usual. A *little
crazy*.... with.... boredom. This always happens after an
exciting little venture out of the house. *Always........
always.... always.* My mind is spinning behind droopy
eyelids. I'm drunk with boredom. Drunk, but not falling
about laughing. Bored.... bored.... bored.... but... just...
too... exhausted... to... do... anything... but... stare... at...
the... wall... or... ceiling. My... body... wants... to... lie...
still. Very... still. Still as a stone. Or a statue. No. Not a
stone or a statue, that sounds too depressing. Still as a
deserted sandy beach on hot summer day in Cornwall,
with the tide gently ebbing and flowing. In.... out.... in....
out. With every inward breath, I breath in a little life.
With every outward breath...... the.... life.... escapes...
me. Blue waves of tiredness wash over me..... wash.....
wash..... wash..... Do I feel some verse coming on? No.
Not today. Today, in my mind's little eye, I will lie on a
sandy beach opposite my house on the Cornish coast,
next door to Dawn French. Then later I will enjoy watching
my cats groom themselves..... groom..... groom..... groom.

3.00 p.m.   Oh God. *Oh God! Oh God! Oh God!* Much as I *love* the
peace of living in our little street. And much as I *love*
lying in my warm comfortable bed, or dozing on the sofa
under a warm blanket of cats, I want to be in London's
West End again. The bright lights. The busy traffic. People
going about their business. Bill Bailey *live.* It all makes me
feel *so alive.* And I forget about me. I forget about M.E.,
and become part of this bright whirlpool of life.

4.00 p.m.   Too tired to read, watch TV, or reply to pen-friends. But
I can stroke my cats. One stroke each. Feel so hungry.
Tummy is rumbling. No energy to make a sandwich. Must
eat something. There's a banana in the fruit bowl with
my name on it. Well, it hasn't actually got my name on
it, but I will find a biro that doesn't work and write my my
name on the skin. The impression will turn a nice shade of
brown, like H.P. sauce (this looks good on banana yellow)
and will be my entertainment for the day. It's the one time

a dead biro is useful, unless you like making sculptures out of melted biros or something.

4.05 p.m. Eat banana, to *hopefully* give me slow burning energy. Stare at can in cupboard, and visualise self full of beans.

5.00 p.m. I fancy a mug of strong coffee to perk me up, but anyone who has M.E. knows this is a *very* bad idea. I will ignore desperate coffee cravings. I will remind myself that coffee is just a hot drink made from the seeds of a tropical shrub. Coffee is a shrub. I would be drinking ground shrub. *Shrub, shrub, shrub.* Will drink de-caf tea instead because it's *much, much, much,* better for me. I will forget that tea is dried leaves of an Asian shrub.

5.05 p.m. Half fill kettle with water.... switch kettle on.... pick a Kit-Kat mug from the mug tree and place on work surface.... rest.... ignore craving for a bar of Kit-Kat.... take lid off tea caddy and take out tea bag.... replace lid.... pop tea bag into mug.... open fridge door and take out a carton of soya milk.... close fridge door and place carton on work surface.... sigh (with a face like Woody Allen suffering from stomach ache).... lift kettle and pour boiling water into mug, until it's three quarters full.... pick up soya milk carton and pour milk into mug, almost to the brim.... rest.... find a teaspoon and take tea-bag out of mug.... place tea bag on small (teapot shaped) used-tea-bag holder.... sit down and slurp, feeling like I've done a hard day's work.... I fancy a slice of hot buttered wholemeal toast.... I wish the fairies would pop in and look after me.

5.35 p.m. I have found some energy to open the fridge door.... take out loaf of Hovis wholemeal bread and tub of Flora margarine.... place loaf and tub on work surface.... take slice of bread out of bag and place in toaster.... find knife and tea plate and place them on work surface.... rest (with a face like Clint Eastwood sulking) while waiting for toast to pop up out of toaster............................ POP!.... remove slice of toast from toaster.... too tired to

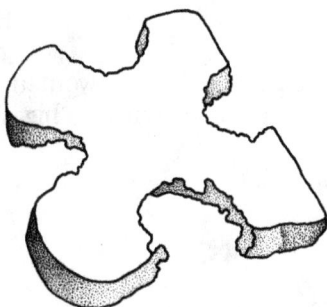

pick up knife and dip into margarine.... pick up toast and bite round the edges (four bites) so it looks a little like a jigsaw puzzle piece.... decide to eat the rest later.... have run out of energy to munch.... lie on sofa cuddling Mary and entertain myself with a daydream.......... I imagine myself biting round the edges of six slices of toast, so they resemble jigsaw puzzle pieces that will fit together. Then spreading all six slices with margarine, each one with a different topping: strawberry jam, lime marmalade, lemon curd, chocolate spread, raspberry jam and orange marmalade (for a tasty colourful puzzle).

6.00 p.m.   Feeling hungry. And bored. Pick up a felt tip pen, then draw on my fingers and toes.

6.20 p.m.

ME: Do you like my funny feet?

BEN: You've written letters on your toes with felt pen, is that funny?

ME: Yes, the letters T, O, M and A.

BEN: Mmm (blank look).

ME: Tomatoes!

BEN: *What are you like.*

ME: Look, I've written F, I, S and H on my fingers.

BEN: Ah, I get that. Crazy woman. I'll come home tomorrow and you'll have written a big number four on your head.

ME: Good idea!

Friday 19th

10.46 a.m.   I texted Ben:

I-M STILL TOO EXHAUSTED TO PREPARE DINS - CAN GET A HIGGIDY QUICHE, I CAN JUST POP IT IN THE OVEN - OH, CAN U GET SUM PREPARED SALAD TOO?

10.48 a.m.   Ben replied:

OK X

10.49 a.m.   GREAT - THANX X

2.15 p.m.   Text message from Jayne:

HOW R U TODAY WITCHY FRIEND?

2.16 p.m.   I replied:

STILL A WORN OUT WITCH - DOIN NUTHIN - HOW R U?

2.18 p.m.   SAME AS YOU X

3.00 p.m.   I stared out of the kitchen window. Leaves were breaking free from tree branches, in a huge gust of wind. I enjoyed watching them pirouette and somersault high into the air, across mother nature's stage. Next door's holly bushes bounced from side to side, laden with red berries, like an excited audience at a pop concert. Ivy leaves flapped and clapped wildly, like an appreciative audience at a comedy show. Who needs London's West End, when you have your own little theatre.

MOTHER NATURE'S STAGE

Act 1   The tree branches are almost bare, just the odd leaf clinging on, here and there. Two squirrels enter stage left, bouncing through the tufts of grass on the lawn. Then they dig furiously to bury the nuts held in their bulging cheeks; rummaging through the piles of pale yellow and brown leaves, like two old ladies at a jumble sale. When their stash is safely buried, they sit upright like tiny meerkats, tails twitching, checking for cats.

Act 2   The stage darkens as rain clouds gather. Thunder rumbles in the distance. It starts to rain and the squirrels hurriedly exit stage right. The scenery is dark gloomy greens. The pale leaves on the lawn are now shiny dark browns and deep yellows. Hedgehogs snore happily with the fairies at the bottom of the garden. A fox enters stage left and takes refuge in the tumble-down garden shed.

Act 3   The rain has stopped and the squirrels return, stage right, to bury more nuts. A large ginger and white cat enters stage left. He leaps from a fence onto the roof of the garden shed, then sits hunched, watching the squirrels with a very still, very silent, fat cat stare. The squirrels ignore him.

Act 4   It's starting to get dark and a waning moon appears. The squirrels have gone home. The cat gets up, yawns and stretches, jumps down from the garden shed, and wanders off, stage right. The odd leaf still flutters in the breeze. The fairies at the bottom of the garden sigh, and flutter their eyelashes in their sleep.

The stage curtains close.

* * * * * *

4.15 p.m.   Doing nothing.
I close the sitting room curtains and lay on the sofa under a blanket of warm cats, listening to *Midsomer Murders: Beyond the grave.* The villagers of Aspern Tallow begin to believe the ghost of a former resident has come back to haunt them..... ooh.... nice and spooky.

6.10 p.m.   Still doing nothing.
Ben isn't home from Sainsbury's yet. Stare out of bedroom window before closing the curtains. Neighbouring houses look dark, but soon there will be Christmas lights twinkling in windows. Who needs London's West End, when you have Christmas fairy lights to look forward to.

> *One of the lessons in history is that nothing is often a good thing to do and always a clever thing to say.*
>
> *WILL DURANT*

Saturday 20th

I felt a little better today, less grey and exhausted and melancholy blue. And although I have my own little theatre in the garden, and the bright lights of Christmas to look forward to, I still wanted to see Bill Bailey again. So I put on one of his DVDs *(Part Troll, Live at the Hammersmith Apollo 2004)* and informed Ben that Bill's next DVD *(Dandelion Mind, Live from Dublin)* will be out on Monday. It will soon be Christmas. Hint, hint.

Bill (best mate Bill) rang Ben on his mobile phone. Bill's voice is so loud, I could hear every word. Not that I was being nosey. No. *Of course not.* I was just passing. Close by. Needed a little entertainment.

BILL: I'm in town today, fancy a drink down The Flowerpot?

BEN: Yeah, OK mate, what time?

BILL: About one?

BEN: Yeah, fine, see you there mate.

BILL: What've you been up to?

BEN: I had two posh birds this morning.

BILL: Great, what were they like?

BEN: Very tasty *and* rich.

BILL: Lucky you.

BEN: Would you like to try some?

BILL: Yeah!

BEN: OK, I'll bring half a dozen down the pub.

BILL: *Cheers mate!*

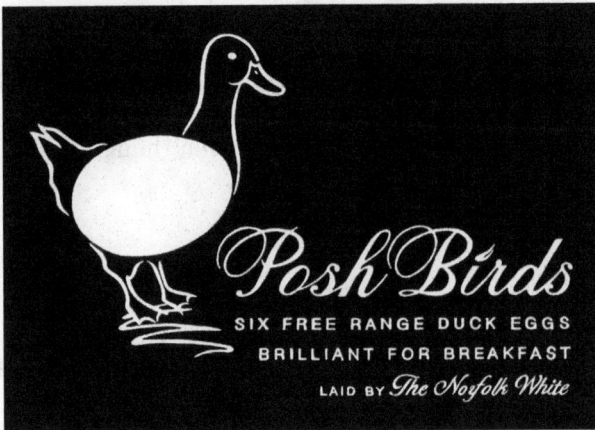

Sunday 21st

ME: These duck eggs are *very* tasty.

BEN: Yeah, and rich.

ME: I hope Bill enjoys 'em.

BEN: He will, he likes a nice posh bird.

ME: There's a double-page spread of posh Advent calendars in Weekly Wife; they're made from wood, felt and cotton. Here, have a look.... lovely bright reds and greens.

BEN: Not as lovely as *your* double-page spread in InterAction.

ME: I agree! Can you buy me an Advent calendar today when you're in town.

BEN: OK, would you like one with chocolates in the little windows?

ME: *Ooh*, yes please, I've *never* had one of *those*.

* * * * * * *

I was passing by Ben's computer tonight when he was busy sending emails. I wasn't being nosey. No. *Nooooo. Of course not.* I just needed a little entertainment, even though I didn't understand a word I read.

Hi Ben,

What is your opinion of Sound Forge 6?
Is there something better?
Thanks for the info – we really have to talk again about compression/exciters and mastering processes.

The soundcard rocks by the way.

NICE ONE!

Rupe.

****

As far as I can see Soundforge is the USA's version of Wavelab. Both are essentially Stereo Mastering programs, Wavelab also has it's "Montage" element which is a kind of multi-track facility but more aimed at Multimedia/Composite projects. I don't know if Soundforge has an equivalent function.

CD burning used to be a bolt-on extra for Soundforge called "CD Architect" whereas it's built into Wavelab – that might not be the case anymore though.
I don't think there is much to choose really in terms of wave file editing, although most reviews do seem to favour Wavelab (in European mags though!)

I guess the bottom line is, if you already know Wavelab then not much point learning another one...

Sonic Foundry do make a great Noise Reduction DX Plugin though... have attached.

Ben.

Monday 22nd

My Monday morning blues were a darker blue than usual. A Prussian blue. Like the sky in Van Gogh's depressing painting, *Starry Night Over the Rhone*. My Monday morning boiled egg was a miserable yellow, like the yellow in Van Gogh's painting, *The Yellow House*. The greens in our garden, reminded me of the sad, mouldy greens in Van Gogh's painting, *View of Arles*. I can't say I'm a fan of any of his work, his paintings make me want to cut both my ears off. Sorry Vincent.

I was tempted to open *all* the little windows in my Advent calendar. Then sinfully eat *all* the little chocolates, one by one. I knew this would *greatly* cheer me up (not just because chocolate makes me feel better) but because I *like* the pictures in Advent windows. *And* I really wanted to know if the chocolates would be festive shapes - a cracker, Christmas tree, or a Christmas pudding.

Instead, I sat gazing at the colourful picture of a jolly Santa on his sleigh (full of presents) with his jolly reindeer. The scene was frosted here and there with silver glitter, and made me feel *jolly Christmassy.*

Strength is the capacity to break a chocolate bar into four pieces with your bare hands - and then eat just one piece.

JUDITH VIORST

Strength is the capacity to gaze at a chocolate Advent calendar and not eat one chocolate ~ until December 1st.

&

Strength is the capacity to cope with the incapacity of M.E.

&

Strength is the capacity not to strangle a rude doctor at an incapacity benefit interview.

&

Strength is smiling and saying nothing, when someone tells you how well you look.

VERITY RED

November

My sad green, miserable yellow, and Prussian Monday morning blues, were lifted when Interflora knocked on the front door just after 10 a.m. Bright cherry red and lemony yellow rosebuds greeted me, in a berry blue basket. They were from my aunt and uncle in Yorkshire, congratulating me on my book, *Love & Best Witches.* I sniffed the scent of the flowers, then sniffed again as happy tears of gratitude blossomed in my eyes.

> *People from a planet without*
> *flowers would think we must be*
> *mad with joy the whole time to*
> *have these things about us.*
>
> *IRIS MURDOCH*

When the post arrived late morning, there was another most welcome surprise; a card from auntie and uncle. The picture on the front was a cute elephant painting the word *Congratulations* in rainbow colours. When did I start using the word cute? I think I caught it off my niece, like I've caught other expressions from younger friends. For example, *I've just had a wake-up-call* and *now I see the bigger picture.* Wake-up-call? To me, a wake-up-call is what you get in a hotel when you want reception to ring you at 8.30 a.m. Seeing the bigger picture, is a trip to the cinema. Or the *pictures,* as we used to call them.

The message inside the card was *cool.* Yes, another word I've caught from my little niece. She said (my aunt, not my niece) my book was a fun read, it made her giggle, and she's going to order some copies for Christmas presents. That's *really cool!*

Tuesday 23rd

10.10 a.m.   I am strong. I am not opening an Advent calendar window. Even though I'm *very* tempted.

10.12 a.m.   I am strong. I am not going to eat an Advent calendar chocolate. Even though I'm *extremely* tempted.

11.00 a.m.   I am strong. I will not sniff the Advent calendar, to see if I can smell the aroma of Cadbury's.

207

11.01 a.m.   I will sniff flowers instead.

11.02 a.m.   I admire my blue basket of cherry red and lemon yellow rosebuds.

11.10 a.m.   I admire the cherry red cherries, and lemon yellow pineapple foam stickers on the fridge door. I think I will find the white fruit bowl.

11.35 a.m.   The green, purple, yellow, red, and orange stickers look great on the fruit bowl. My Tuesday morning blues have lifted.

1.33 p.m.   I love the hearth candle holder (with lots of curly bits) in Scots of Stow gift catalogue. I can imagine curly smoke whisping out of the candle flames. The ivory pillar Advent calendar candle looks lovely too, but *not* as *lovely* as an Advent calendar full of little chocolates.

1.36 p.m.   I *will not* feel tempted to open a calendar window, but I *am* tempted to order the curly hearth candle holder, and the happy cat tea-light holder.

Man loves company ~
even if it is only that
of a small burning
candle.

G. C. LICHTENBERG

4.30 p.m.   Ben sent a text message:

GOIN 2 GIG STRAIT FROM WORK 2NITE X

A girl loves company ~
even if it is only that
of a small text
message.

VERITY RED

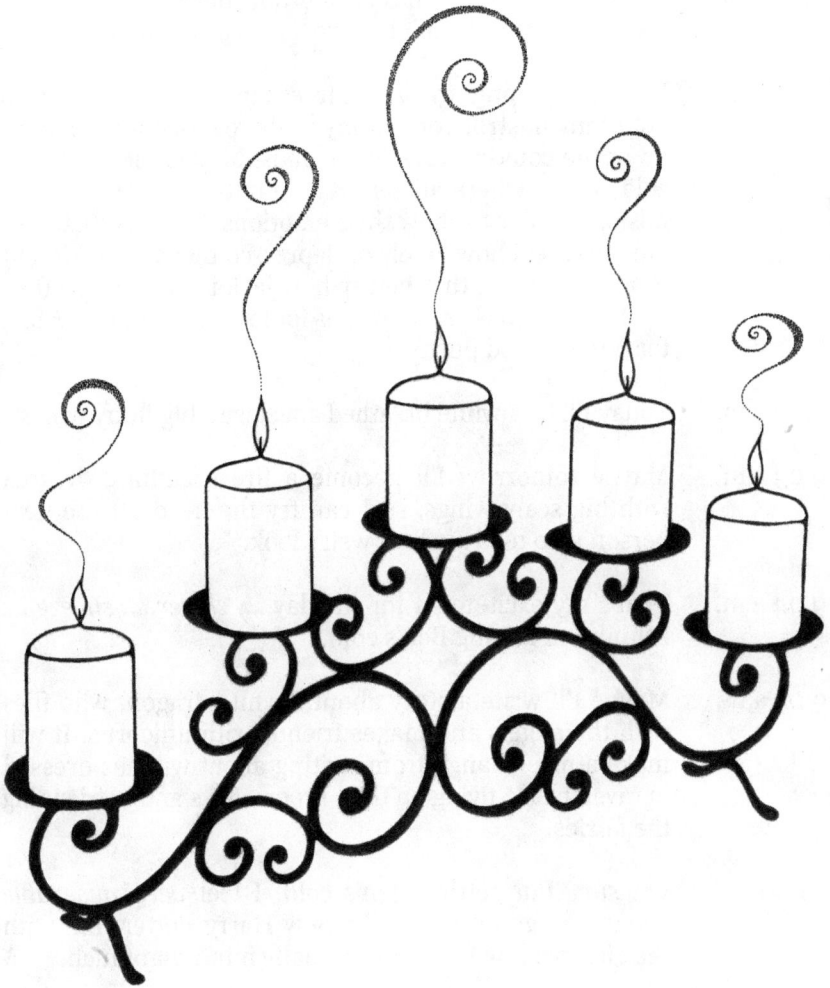

Wednesday 24th

8.57 a.m.   I wrap-up warm to feed the wildlife.

8.59 a.m.   The sky is full of Wednesday morning blues, couldn't-care-less clouds, and I can't believe how *icy cold* it is.

9.00 a.m.   I enjoy watching my breath freeze in a mist, as it billows out of my nostrils (or is it my brain fog escaping). I stare up at the couldn't-care-less clouds. Maybe there's an icy cold planet where aliens breathe out different coloured mists, in order to show their emotions. Various shades of blue to reveal how lonely or depressed they feel. Different shades of green, that betray how jealous or envious they are feeling. Pinks and crimsons for love and passion. White for honesty and purity.

9.02 a.m.   Today I'll be a white breathed angel with big fluffy wings.

9.03 a.m.   Maybe tomorrow I'll become a fire breathing dragon, with big scaly wings, so I can fry the head off the next person who tells me how well I look.

9.04 a.m.   That's my excitement for the day..... *shiver*..... *sneeze*..... I think I'm getting Ben's cold.

9.05 a.m.   Maybe I'll write a story about a white dragon, who flies with the angels and makes friends with unicorns. It will make a nice change from writing about witches dressed in raven black, flying on their broomsticks and befriending the fairies.

10.00 a.m.   I'm *sure* I'm getting Ben's cold, I feel *very miserable* about him going to see the new Harry Potter film with the girls from work. I don't usually mind that much.

10.01 a.m.   He'll be with five young attractive wimmen (a spelling I prefer). Five full of life and laughter females, wearing fashionably-flirty clothes.

10.02 a.m.   I'm breathing out five deep purpley-blue mists, and ten snotty-green shades of envy.

10.03 a.m.   The film looks *really* good, I've seen some extracts on TV. I hope Ben sneezes big-man-germs all over the girls from work *and* their popcorn, *and* they catch all his germs. Or, I hope they are unsuitably dressed for this freezing weather, and catch a chill on the walk from the car park to the cinema. I'm not a very nice person today.

> *There is no such thing as bad weather, only inappropriate clothing.*
>
> *SIR RANULPH FIENNES*

Thursday 25th

10.30 a.m.   Reading Weekly Wife.

10.37 a.m.   Katy Perry has launched her first fragrance, Purr eau de parfum. It's a fresh floral scent, with rich tones of vanilla orchid and sandalwood, in a glass cat-shaped bottle. She designed it herself. *Lucky Katy*, her very own purr-fume.

10.38 a.m.   I hope her perfume makes her sneeze. I'm still not a very nice person today, my head full of Thursday morning blues.

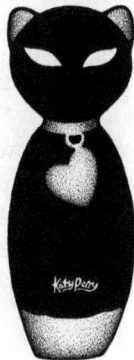

10.43 a.m.   How weird! I've just read an article about a man named Dominic Zenden, and discovered there *really is* a planet where the beings breath out colours. It's our planet, Earth!

Dominic sees human auras. He says the best way to describe an aura is that there's this three-dimensional cloud surrounding everyone, and it contains a flow of colours that are constantly mingling and moving. These flows change according to a person's mood. Then he goes on to say he can't remember a time when he *couldn't* see them. It was just part of his world, and he came to realise that these colours represented what people were thinking and feeling. He continues.....

I used to think of my grandmother as the 'green lady' because whenever she spoke, she was surrounded by shades of green. I now know that eating a lot of sugar and smoking cigarettes creates a green colour. My father was quite an aggressive man, and if he raised his voice, puffs of red would come out of his mouth. I saw the same from a teacher at school who shouted a lot.
At first you don't know what the colours mean, but knowledge builds over the years. You learn to associate colours with particular emotions.

How strange and fascinating!

6.30 p.m.   Feel flu-ish and wobbly. Miserable as Van Gogh in *all* his thirty self portraits. I want to eat *all* the chocolates in my Advent calendar. I wonder if my aura is shades of grey-blue.

7.30 p.m.   *Coronation Street* is wonderfully miserable. Kevin tries to convince Molly not to reveal their secret.

8.30 p.m.   More *Coronation Street*. John gets a shock when the identity of his stalker is finally revealed.

9.00 p.m.

ME: Can you hide the Advent calendar from me.

BEN: Yes dear.

Friday 26th

A pack of children's birthday cards and birthday gift wrap arrived from ACE catalogue today. I liked the cupcake pictures (especially the cupcake fairy) but felt too ill to enjoy all pastel coloured designs. I couldn't even manage half a smile, but I could have managed a cupcake with a nice cuppa.

I spent most of the day sleeping or cloud watching. Cloud watching can be very therapeutic if you use a little imagination..... a Scotty dog..... with a dragon's tail..... the tail grows longer..... the arrow shaped end of the tail breaks off..... slowly floats away..... followed by a cupcake..... the cake flattens and becomes a currant bun..... followed by an elephant..... with a small trunk..... the trunk grows longer and turns into a scorpion's tail..... the elephant's head is now a mole..... followed by a sleeping bear..... I fall asleep..... I dream of fluffy pink and white cupcakes, sprinkled with silvery stars..... floating in a sky of Friday blues.

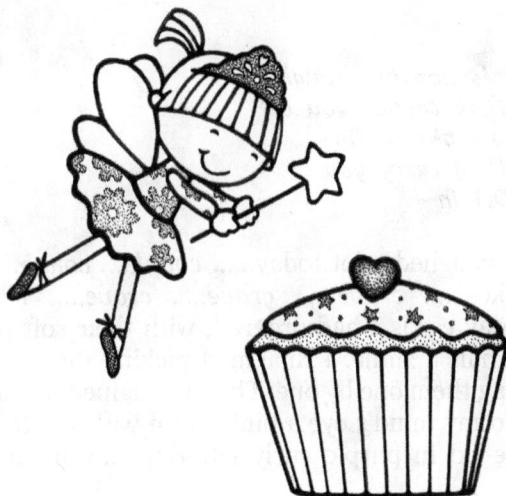

Saturday 27th

I woke up barely able to breathe, and I couldn't speak at all because my chest was so tight. The inhaler I hadn't used for years was out of date, so Ben got a prescription from an emergency doctor for a new one. While I waited for him to collect it, I really *did* feel I might die. I had recently seen a novelty red and white Kit-Kat coffin gift in a catalogue (*Death by Chocolate* written on the side) and decided that when I die, I would like a coffin exactly the same.

Ben was my knight with the shiny inhaler that saved my life; and although I felt lucky to be alive, I thought about a red and white Kit-Kat coffin. I liked the thought of relatives smiling at my funeral, everyone dressed in red and white, instead of mournful black. Maybe I'll write that in my will.

6.26 p.m.   Text message from Ben:

POPPING INTO TESCO FOR SUM BEERS ON MY WAY HOME FROM BILL'S , DO U WANT ANYTHING?

6.28 p.m.   I replied:

GARLIC, ORANGES, AND A KIT-KAT - THANX X

Sunday 28th

It's not the coughin'
That carries you off
It's the coffin
They carry you
Off in

I coughed a lot today...... *cough....* *cough.....* *cough.....* I craved cupcakes...... *crave......* *crave.....* *crave.....* I admired the cupcake birthday cards I had ordered, with their soft pastel shades, and managed half a smile. I imagined picking the cakes out of the cards and eating them one by one. Then I imagined feeling ill. Very ill. I died. I saw in my mind's eye a pink coffin with *Death by Cupcakes* written on the lid in purple curly lettering; my mourners wearing pink, white, pastel blues and greens, and eating cupcakes after the funeral. Cupcakes with a theme. I *love* cupcakes with a theme. Like Halloween. I saw black and orange cupcakes with pumpkin and spider web design, advertised in Weekly Wife last month. Very tempting. A celebrity (also in Weekly Wife) can't recall her name (one of those girl bands where they all look the same) had a baby shower, where the cupcake theme was Alice in Wonderland. *Wonderful!* The icing was bright Disney colours. Am I rambling on about cupcakes? I can't help it........... I must be a little delirious....... *cough...... cough...... cough......* Where was I?............ Oh yes! I was at Weekly Wife's Wonderland photo shoot. I recall, some of the cakes with swirly turquoise icing and a tiny white playing card (red Ace card design) neatly placed on top. There were miniature orange and blue teapots and teacups on doilies, and flowers sitting on grass green swirls too. But my favourite design was the Cheshire Cats (*no surprise there*, I hear you think) with pink and purple stripy smiley faces. My niece loved the owl cake I had made for her birthday, with ten baby owl cupcakes (Smarties for eyes) to match. Her birthday party was a real hoot. I'd like a chocolate cat cake for my funeral...... *cough..... cough...... cough......* (death day party) and cupcakes with paw prints on. Cupcakes the colour of all the cats I've cared for: black, ginger, grey, and shades of brown. The paw prints could be white icing. It's such a lovely idea, I think I may treat myself next birthday, because when I'm dead, I don't want to be floating around craving chocolate cake (and listening to what people are saying about me) wishing I'd enjoyed cupcakes with a *theme* when I was alive.

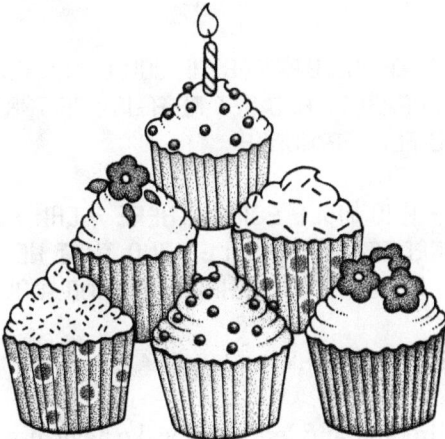

In this week's Weekly Wife, the thin models (I'll bet they've never tasted a cupcake) were dancing around with big smiles, shiny eyes and glossy hair. They jumped for joy in this season's jumper dresses, pattered around in patterned tights, and looked gorgeous in georgette style blouses. I plodded around, with watery eyes and greasy hair, wearing my old black dressing gown, with pink paw print design. I knew a nice little cupcake would make my eyes shine, and my taste buds dance with joy.

2.30 p.m.   Text message from Ben:

POPPING INTO SAINS-B ON WAY HOME FROM ALEX-S, DO U WANT ANYTHING?

2.31 p.m.   I replied:

CUPCAKES – THANX X

2.32 p.m.   OK

2.33 p.m.   OH – AND SOYA MILK

2.35 p.m.   AND TISSUES

2.36 p.m.   YES DEAR – ANYTHING ELSE ?

2.37 p.m.   WELL, IT WUD BE GREAT IF YOU COULD POP INTO HOLLAND AND BARRETT AND GET ME A JAR OF THAT LUVLI ORGANIC WILD FLOWER HONEY

2.38 p.m.   OH – AND WHILE YOR IN THERE – CAN YOU GET EVENING PRIMROSE OIL CAPSULES AND THAT HERB TEA – SNORE AND PEACE – WITH CHAMOMILE AND LAVENDER ?

2.40 p.m.   CERTAINLY DEAR

5.00 p.m.   I'm in pink and lemon cupcake heaven.

5.01 p.m.	My taste buds are dancing with joy.
5.02 p.m.	My eyes are shining.
5.15 p.m.	My throat is soothed with organic wild flower honey.
5.30 p.m.	My mouth is smiling. A *wide* smile. I'm admiring the kitchen roll Ben has bought. We have three rolls in the kitchen cupboard, but he thought the colourful cupcake design would cheer me up too. *It does!*

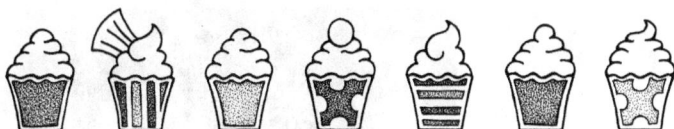

7.00 p.m.	I notice our street is sprinkled with a fine layer of snow.
7.15 p.m.	I'm sitting peacefully at my bedroom window, watching the snow sparkle on car bonnets, like tiny silvery stars on white cupcakes.
7.25 p.m.	I'm sipping herbal tea with chamomile, lemon balm, and honey.
8.15 p.m.	I'm snoring in peace.
8.30 p.m.	I'm dreaming of a plate of white cupcakes, tiny silver star shapes falling through the air, to land artily on white icing, like constellations in the night sky.
8.31 p.m.	Cupcake fairies flutter in a cosmic way around my head.
9.00 p.m.	I'm dreaming of lying in bed at night with the curtains open, watching snowflakes silently fall.
9.01 p.m.	I hear the sound of sleigh bells in the distance.
9.05 p.m.	I'm dreaming of a white Christmas.

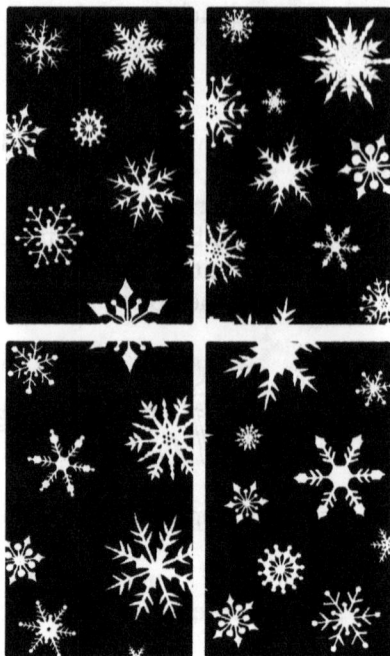

Monday 29th

NOVEMBER COLD

Cough, sneeze
Cough, sneeze
The garden is
A deep freeze

Cough, sneeze
Cough, sneeze
November skies
November breeze

Cough, sneeze
Cough, sneeze
November chills
November trees

218

November

Cough, Sneeze
Cough, Sneeze
Feeling wobbly
At the knees

Cough, Sneeze
Cough, Sneeze
I'll have another
Lemsip please

✳

When I get a cold, I like strong and absorbent kitchen roll with thirst pockets and a cheerful pattern. When my nose becomes red and sore, I *love* soft velvety tissue with a soothing aloe vera and camomile balm. If we haven't got either, and I start a cold after shopping night in the week, I make do with Tesco toilet roll until the weekend.

Luckily Ben had bought three rolls of strong and absorbent kitchen roll on Saturday. The packaging said it had thirst pockets as strong as an elephant, because elephants can hold as much as two gallons of water in their trunks at any one time. This is useful when you have a streaming cold, because you feel like you have two gallons of water pouring out of your nose.

There were delightful, colourful pictures of Winnie-the-Pooh all over the kitchen roll. Pooh bear with his honey pot. Pooh bear chasing bees. Pooh bear sitting next to his honey pot, paws covered with honey. This brightened my day and made me smile, because I'm a *big fan* of Winnie-the-Pooh and his adventures with Tigger, Owl, Piglet, Rabbit, Kanga, Roo and Christopher Robin.

I decided to cheer myself up by finding my copy of *The Complete Winnie-the-Pooh,* containing *Winnie-the-Pooh* and *The House at Pooh Corner* by the wonderful A.A. Milne, fantastically illustrated by E. H. Shephard. I flicked through the pages to find my favourite Pooh poem before I started reading the first book.

LINES WRITTEN BY A BEAR OF VERY LITTLE BRAIN

On Monday, when the sun is hot
I wonder to myself a lot:
'Now is it true, or is it not,
That what is which and which is what?'

On Tuesday, when it hails and snows,
The feeling on me grows and grows
That hardly anybody knows
If those are these or these are those.

On Wednesday, when the sky is blue,
And I have nothing else to do,
I sometimes wonder if it's true
That who is what and what is who.

On Thursday, when it starts to freeze
And hoar~frost tinkles on the trees,
How very readily one sees
That those are whose ~ but whose are these?

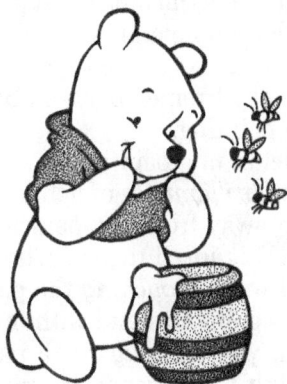

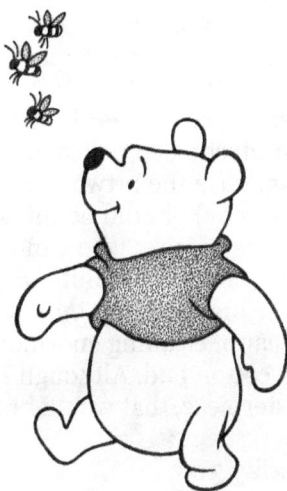

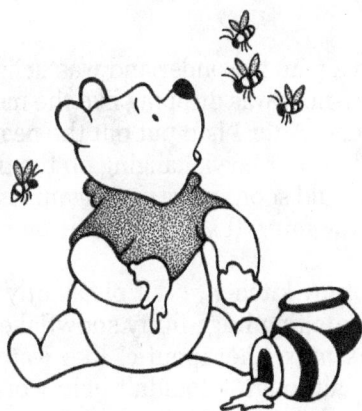

I cackled quietly to myself as I read the poem, then sneezed into a big strong sheet of kitchen roll (with wonderful little thirst pockets). It seemed a pity to blow my nose on such pretty pictures of Pooh bear, and I recalled a day I visited London's Tate Gallery (one of many visits in my art student days). This particular day I remember well because I got told off. My nose was too close to a painting.

I had been admiring the detail in a painting of a vase of flowers. Such *amazing* use of colour. Such *brilliant* use of light. Such..... a policeman-type-voice told me to step away from the painting, my nose was a few inches from the canvas. I ignored the security-type-person and wandered off. Stupid man. I wasn't *touching* the painting with my hands. Did he *really* think I was going to stand with my nose *actually* touching the masterpiece? Can you *actually see* a painting with your nose stuck to it? Did he think I was trying to *smell* the flowers? Had he ever bothered to appreciate any of the paintings he was protecting so policemanly-protectively? Did he think I was going to *vandalise* the artwork with my nose? OK, my nose is a bit *pointy* (and witchy) but did he think it would actually *cut* the canvas? Maybe there *are* witches who can cut things with their pointy noses, if they put their mind to it. But that's beside the *point*. I should have sneezed all over the painting, *that* would have got me arrested and sentenced to a year of cleaning enormous, old, tobacco stained oil paintings with a tiny cotton bud. Although I would *never, ever* dream of sneezing on a masterpiece, that would be sacrilege.

Tuesday 30ᵗʰ

Feeding the wildlife in a winter wonderland was delightful today, even though my pointy-witchy-nose was dripping like the melting snow on the leaves of our privet hedge. After I had put out the peanuts, I poured hot water into the little fairy water bowl, hanging on the trellis. The ice melted away, but I knew it would soon freeze over again, and I'd have to do what I call, de-frosting the fairy. It's a chore, but more fun than de-frosting the fridge.

Back in the warmth of my kitchen, I felt pleasantly calm and soothed, as I sipped Lemsip, watching huge fluffy snowflakes fall through Lemsipy steam. This was *most* therapeutic, like watching fluffy clouds sail across a blue sky; although I couldn't help worrying that Ben might not get home safely from work. I decided to text him, telling him there was heavy snowfall in this part of the country, and maybe he should leave work early.

Late morning I felt lonely and low, and wondered if I should wrap-up and stand outside in the snow, pretending I'm in a pretty snow globe. That would cheer me up, but probably leave me feeling a little shaken, with white spots before my eyes. I de-frosted the fairy, then thought I may start writing Christmas cards. I enjoy writing Christmas cards. I *love* the satisfaction of seeing a nice big pile of crisp white envelopes, neatly addressed and stamped with a jolly Christmas stamp. Some years (if I have the energy) I like to draw a holly design on the envelopes with red and green felt tip pens, and tie the small piles of cards up with festive gold ribbon. Then I can rest, admiring a job *well done*; while the snow lies deep and crisp and even, and there's a deep-pan, crisp and even pizza in the oven, the mozzarella cheese bubbling like excited children on a *Merry Christmas* morning.

My nose continued to drip like a plumber's nightmare, so I decided that it wasn't a good idea to start writing cards and envelopes. But I *had* to do *something*.

11.30 a.m. Found my Disney jigsaw puzzle. Completed Snow White and one of the seven dwarves, Sneezy.

2.00 p.m. Ben sent a text message:

LEAVING SOON DUE TO SNOW, WILL BE IN CONVOY WITH ROB SO NO WORRIES X

2.01 p.m. I replied:

OH, THAT-S GOOD — SAFE JOURNEY HOME X

*An avalanche begins with
a snowflake*

JOSEPH COMPTON

Chapter
Five

December

Today the garden slept peacefully and serenely under a thick, lumpy white quilt. I spent most of the day, peacefully and serenely sleeping under a thick flowery quilt, content in the knowledge that I had survived another year. Well, almost a whole year, just a few weeks to go.

It was supposed to be an exciting day; opening my first Advent calendar window, writing my first Christmas cards, maybe putting up the odd Christmas decoration, or writing a Christmas letter. I dreamt about it all instead. Much less tiring.

Zzzzzzzzzzzz

Early evening, I opened a square Advent Calendar window with a number one on it. I couldn't see the *one* at first because I had sleepy M.E. eyeballs, but I finally found it on a reindeer's hoof. I was greeted by a smiling teddy bear on a Cadbury's purple background. He wore an emerald green bow around his neck, and held a red and white candy stick. I thought the piece of chocolate might be a little plain square, but I was delighted to find it was the shape of a cracker. I bit the end off the cracker. It snapped beautifully, then melted on my tongue, like snow in winter sunshine. That was my excitement for the day.

Thursday 2nd

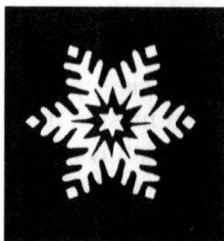

I opened an Advent calendar window before my first sneeze of the day. Finding the tiny number two on a reindeer's antler was my first challenge of the day. The picture was a white snowflake on a purple Cadbury's background. The chocolate was snowflake shaped, and dissolved on my tongue, like a snowflake settling on the warm nose of a human with a cold. My second challenge of the day was to *not* open the rest of the windows and eat *all* the chocolates.

The garden slept snugly under two thick white quilts of snow. I was a red nose reindeer hiding in my warm stable, snuffling around for something tasty to nibble. Ben had to work from home (because of the snow) so he was my stable mate, tapping his hooves on computer keys, and occasionally foraging for food.

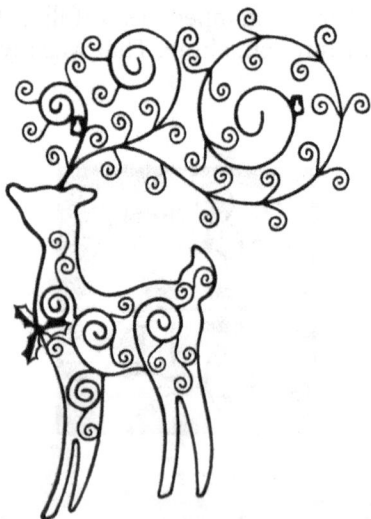

December

I noticed a reindeer shaped card holder in a Christmas catalogue; I liked the design, especially the big curly antlers. I decided to order it, because our shelves are crammed with so many ornaments, there's barely any room for cards. There was a choice of gold or silver. I chose the gold, to match the gold tinsel I would eventually get round to draping here and there, in our sitting room.

Early evening, neither reindeer felt like cooking dinner, so they enjoyed having a Chinese meal delivered. Both agreed it was a delicious treat, as they nodded their antlers; munching onions, carrots and mushrooms in a tasty black bean sauce.

Friday 3rd

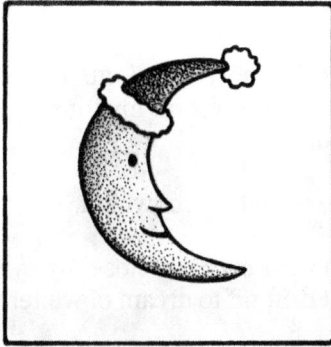

9.45 a.m.   I shuffle through the snow wearing bright red wellies, and carrying extra supplies to the bird table. Feeling washed-out and wobbly as lemon jelly, I try not to fall over. I may not have the energy to get up again.

9.46 a.m.   A robin is bobbing on the fence nearby.

ME: Good morning Bobby.

BOBBY: Hello, I like your red wellies (robin language).

ME: Thanks, they match your chest don't they?

BOBBY: Yes, and your nose! (robin language).

ME: What are you like.

BOBBY: A picture on a Christmas card (robin language).

ME: You're right, and if I had the energy I'd rush indoors, find my camera, and take a photo of you. But I expect by the time I came back you'd have flown away.

BOBBY: Of course!
Oh, and don't forget to de-frost the fairy (robin language).

9.49 a.m.   I droop under the weight of my old denim blue jacket, like the snow laden leaves of our privet hedge, as I shuffle back indoors.

10.00 a.m.   A smiling moon wears a Santa hat in today's window. The chocolate star melts on my tongue, like starlight melting away at dawn.

10.05 a.m.   I feel like a melting snowman.

1.25 p.m.   I curl up with my cats, close my eyes, and the day melts away as I drift off to dream of winter wonderlands, *far, far away*.

6.30 p.m.   Ben puts a fresh pizza in the oven, till the mature cheddar, mascarpone and ricotta cheese melts.

7.30 p.m.   *Coronation Street*. Tonight Nick begs Leanne to marry him. It's *so* romantic, my heart melts like a chocolate heart on a hot radiator.

10.25 p.m.   Before I go to bed I sit watching the snow covered car park opposite our house. No cars. *No* recycling skips. No footprints. Just a beautiful expanse of undisturbed snow illuminated by moonlight. I feel writerly.

10.27 p.m.   Moonbeams gently kiss the evening snow..... like a groom softly kissing his blushing bride in white satin, on their winter wedding day..... The snow sparkles like a million diamonds of joy in her eyes..... happy tears roll down her cheeks..... dripping into snow..... melting into the snow..... and falling..... deeply..... irrevocably..... in pure..... white..... honest..... love.

10.28 p.m.   That was a bit slushy. But my beloved Charles Baudelaire, the poet I should have married in Paris, would have loved those words, uttered from my *beige rosé* lips.

Saturday 4ᵗʰ

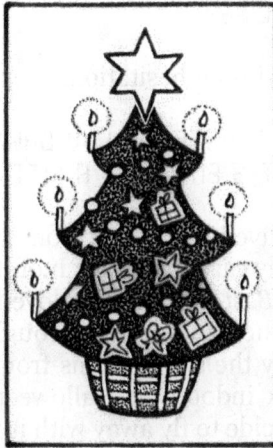

9.15 a.m.   I felt a little better today, after a very romantic night of dreams of being in Paris..... Paris covered in a honeymoon-white quilt of snow..... with Charles.

9.21 a.m.   On my way to fill the bird table, I noticed the seven dwarves garden ornaments were tucked up under a quilt of snow, all I could see were seven small snowy lumps.

SNOW WHITE

Snow all white and lumpy
Sleepy, Happy, Grumpy
Freezing cold and breezy
Dopey, Doc and Sneezy.

9.22 a.m.   I thought I'd better not recite the verse to the dwarves, Bashful might feel left out.

9.30 a.m.   Today's Advent calendar window opened to reveal a Christmas tree draped with decorations. The chocolate holly melted on my tongue, like a chocolate decoration on a Christmas tree, hanging too near a radiator.

9.46 a.m.   Received a text message from my sister:

              HI – CAN-T THINK WOT 2 GET U 4 XMAS – IS THERE A BOOK U-D LIKE?

9.47 a.m.   I replied, without hesitation:

              OH, YES – I-D REALLY LUV DAWN FRENCH-S NEW BOOK – I THINK IT-S ENTITLED, A LITTLE BIT MARVELLOUS X

11.26 a.m.   A letter arrived in the post from Dad. He thanked me for the birthday card I sent last month, enclosed with a copy of *Love & Best Witches*. He loved the book, and said he still uses the broomstick I bought in the seventies, to brush away the snow on his front porch. He brings the broomstick indoors at Halloween in case the trick-or-treaters decide to fly away with it.
              Unlike Uncle Vernon and Aunt Petunia in the Harry Potter films, I think my Dad *is proud* to have a witch in the family!

1.14 p.m.   In Weekly Wife there was a double-page spread of their top ten Christmas Trees – *Whatever your style, budget or room size, we've found a perfect tree for the family.*

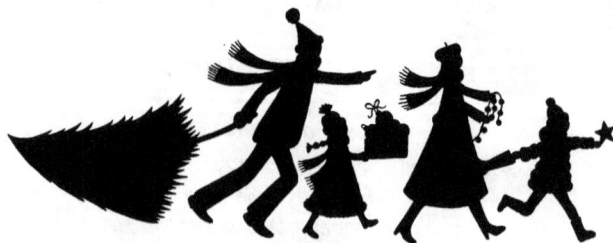

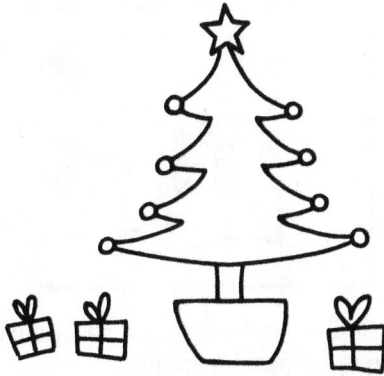

One of the trees was small and wooden, and reminded me of the way my little niece draws Christmas trees; the branches curving upwards, baubles on the ends of the branches, and a big star on top.

On the next page there was an article about Dawn French, mentioning her new book, *A Tiny Bit Marvellous*. I wondered whether to send my sister a text message, telling her I got the title of Dawn's book a tiny bit wrong. Then I decided not to, because it would give her a laugh when she realised my *tiny-but-marvellous* mistake.

Sunday 5th

As I coughed my way to the bird table this morning, I noticed the rain had melted away some of the snow. My seven dwarves were peering out of their fluffy white blankets, and their little faces made me smile. For a moment I felt inspired to complete more of my Disney jigsaw puzzle, but I knew I had to save energy for writing Christmas cards and letters.

Two jolly snowmen greeted me when I opened the window marked with a number five, on Santa's sleigh. The chocolate robin melted on my tongue, like a Cadbury's Flake on a hot summer day. Summer seemed a very long time ago.

Gazing out of the bedroom window mid-afternoon, I saw another snowman in the car park. He was melting and his head had fallen off. I couldn't help thinking that M.E. is like being a snowman after a rainfall. Your energy dissolves away, you feel like you've lost

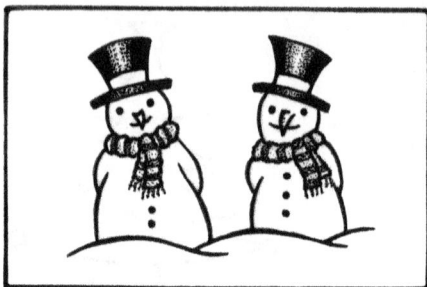

your head; and you end up feeling like a puddle of slush, unable to do anything but gaze up at passing clouds.

3.10 p.m. I did some cloud watching.
A hare with long crinkly ears..... a crocodile with long spindly legs..... a horizontal seahorse..... duck with a horse's tail..... dragon with a cat's head..... a devil's fork..... without a devil..... a snail with short horns..... wolf with the body of a turtle..... a shoe..... a pair of shrews..... a jaguar..... the sort of jaguar with legs and a tail..... a bonnet..... the sort you wear on your head..... a cupid riding on a hedgehog..... a hippo with wings..... an angel on skis...... on skis!

4.05 p.m. I decided, after over seventeen years of cloud watching, I have become an expert. I will award myself a Diploma in cloud watching with a fancy border. Or maybe I'll write a book about a witch who always has her head in the clouds, because she flies too high on her broomstick. She will have exciting adventures; meeting a dragon with a cat's head, a horizontal seahorse, a hippo with wings.....

Good Idea.
I'm tired
of being
down
to
earth.

December

5.10 p.m.

BEN: It's a pity the snowman in the car park has nearly gone.

ME: He's got M.E. His energy is melting away, he's lost his
           head, and soon he'll be a puddle of slush. But he'll remain
           very down to earth!

BEN: Yes dear.

ME: Snowmen are like celebrities.

BEN: Whyzat?

ME: Because when they have a meltdown, they are not a
           pretty sight.

BEN: What are you like.

8.20 p.m.   Ben watched the snooker. I lay on the sofa relaxing to
           the peaceful sound of balls clacking, people clapping,
           and the sound of a running commentary from a deep
           manly voice. I closed my eyes..... *he's taking the pink.....
           ninety five..... he's going for the clearance..... one
           hundred and two.....* (audience clapping)*..... remaining
           seven frames to come.....* (doze)*..... a dangerous shot to
           take on..... red above the black..... a favourable kiss off
           the red puts you nicely on the blue..... the risky shot.....
           it shot to the right..... tremendous shot.....* (doze)*..... the
           red just above the blue..... any harder and that wouldn't
           have gone in..... easy to keep it up..... the pink's a
           possibility.....* (doze)*..... you can see the balls jumping,
           watch.....* (eyes open)*..... instead of getting the full ball
           kiss on the red which meant he'd be absolutely dead
           straight on the pink, I don't know whether he can hold
           it for the red, he may have to go in and out.....*

Monday 6th

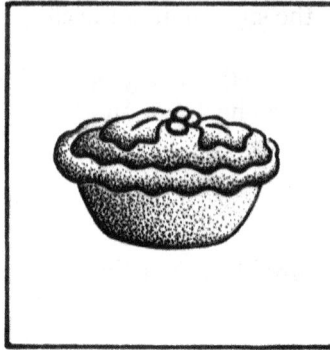

Our first three Christmas cards arrived late morning: a robin on a flowerpot in the snow, a reindeer surrounded by sparkly snowflakes, and Victorian Christmas shoppers in the snow. I felt too weary and achy to start writing Christmas cards, but found the energy to open my Advent calendar window. A mince pie.

1.00 p.m.   I texted Ben:

CAN YOU PUT MINCE PIES ON THE SHOPPIN LIST PLZ ?

1.20 p.m.   Ben replied:

WILL DO X

1.21 p.m.   GOODY – THANX X

Today's chocolate snowman melted away on my tongue, like the snowman in the car park opposite our house. I hoped the children who built him wouldn't be too sad; I always felt a slushy sadness when my beautiful white creation slowly dissolved into the lawn. In my minds eye, I could still see the garden where I played as a child, when my family lived in Chatham. In the winter I loved to build a snowman with my sister. He would have two lumps of coal for his eyes and a carrot nose. He was always a *very groovy* snowman because it was the sixties.

I recall seeing the first man to land on the moon, Neil Armstrong, on our black and white TV too, in the sixties. Scientists can send men in spaceships to land on the moon, but they haven't invented something to stop a snowman melting in your garden.

I started to feel as low as the snowman in the car park. I was just a small lump. Alone. Insignificant. I wanted more snow. Lots more snow. I wanted more energy. Lots more youthful energy, so I could build a big snowman on our lawn, with coal eyes and a carrot nose. We don't use coal for fuel, but there were a few sprouts in the veg rack. I imagined I could paint a couple of them black, with the food colouring I use for monster mash potato at Halloween. They would make perfect snowman eyes. There was an old woody, long and pointy carrot with the potatoes in the veg rack too.

1.30 p.m. I remembered I have a small collection of Christmas cards. Wonderful winter-wonderlandy-woodlandy scenes; with sunshine sparkling on snow, and the odd one with a sprinkling of glitter here and there. I've collected them over the past few years, and will pop them in a clip frame one day. Just gazing at the tranquil photography makes me feel calm and peaceful.

1.32 p.m. Decided to find the cards.

1.35 p.m. Sipped Ben's coffee to perk me up and give me a little energy.

1.40 p.m. Couldn't find the cards. *Anywhere.* But I found all sorts of things I'd forgotten about, and sometimes wondered *where-on-earth-they'd-got-to.*

1.48 p.m. I became engrossed in one of my diaries, written in 2002, when I'd had M.E. for about nine years and was only moderately ill (after many years of being severely ill). I felt very sad reading about people and pets that have since passed away, and I realised how much my health has deteriorated over the past eight years for various reasons. BUT I remain positive about the future, I *know* I *will* make a reasonable recovery again one day.

1.50 p.m.   An entry in the 17th of May made me smile, a sunny smile.

I sat in the garden today. The sun was so hot it felt like summer had finally arrived; she made her entrance smiling brightly, her teeth dazzling white. Everyone warmed to her and smiled back. She positively glowed with appreciation and beamed all day. Her presence was most welcome and everyone hoped she would return tomorrow.

A bumble bee appeared to be nibbling at the tastiest looking flowers, like a guest at a wedding reception buffet. After a brief visit to each colourful bloom, she gave a little buzz of satisfaction. I laughed. She gave me a little buzz too. Then she flew away, and I hoped my witchy cackle hadn't embarrassed her, bees are very sensitive creatures.

A plump lime green caterpillar was enjoying the lemon variegated thyme. I wondered if he would emerge from his chrysalis, a lemon yellow butterfly. He undulated over the herb branches, bringing to mind long carriages full of screaming children, riding along a thin track at a funfair. I gently pulled off a leaf of variegated thyme, careful not to disturb my my tiny green companion. I rubbed it between my thumb and forefinger (the leaf not the caterpillar) although he may have appreciated a little light massage, you never know. I sniffed my finger tip. I breathed in deeply. The best herbal aromatherapy in the world.

On my way indoors for a pepperminty cuppa, I noticed several small snails were sleeping, curled up tight in their shells in a neat row, along the top of our back door. I was reminded of my old cream cardigan with a neat row of small wooden buttons. It certainly wasn't cardie weather today! The sun dried my long witchy hair in no time, like a Babyliss hair dryer on full blast.

Both episodes of *Coronation Street* were exciting tonight. There was an explosion at the joinery, Charlotte pushed John too far, and Molly told Tyrone the truth about Jack. Afterwards I watched the first historic episode shown in 1960, in black and white. ITV were celebrating 50 years of *Coronation Street*. Ken Barlow's round at the

Rovers Return was four shillings and seven pence halfpenny; under thirty pence in today's money!

Watching black and white TV took me back to my childhood again, although I don't recall watching *Coronation Street*. There were no remote controls in those days. I can't imagine watching TV without one now, especially since I got M.E. God bless the remote control.

8.21 p.m.   Received a text message from Jayne. I had texted her last night, telling her Ben had completed my website. There was now music and sound effects, and he had linked her witchy website to mine. Jayne is a very gifted witch who does Tarot readings online, and is writing a review of my witchy book on her website. God bless a good friend!

HEY SUPER WITCHY FRIEND - I TOOK A LOOK AT UR SITE - IT-S SO WONDERFULLY WITCHY - I-M GOING TO HAV THE MUSIC IN MY HEAD ALL DAY - WHICH IS FAB - THANK U SO MUCH FOR ADDING THE LINK TO MY SITE - LOVING WITCH HUG XXX

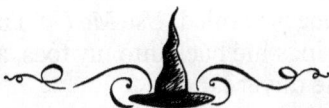

8.47 p.m.   Received a text message from our musician friend Danny. He is a very talented singer/songwriter and guitarist who loves to play the Blues. We haven't seen him play since earlier this year, when he did a gig with his mate Pete at our local pub. The Pilot is close to our house so I don't have far to walk, I mean *stagger* home on Ben's arm. I don't drink much when I go out (*no really!*) but Ben is *hilarious* after a few pints and makes me fall about cackling. Anyway, I had texted Danny last night, to let him know Ben had put a link from my website to his, advertising his music.

www.dannykyle.com

HI VERITY – GREAT TO HEAR FROM YOU – HUGE THANKS
FOR ADDING THE LINK - HOPE TO SEE YOU BOTH
SOMETIME SOON – DANNY X

8.48 p.m.   I replied:

YOU ARE MOST WELCOME DANNY – WE HOPE TO SEE YOU
IN THE NOT TOO DISTANT FUTURE – VERITY X

9.00 p.m.   Decided I needed an early night after a very tiring day hunting for Winter-Wonderlandy Christmas cards and *two* exciting episodes of *Coronation Street*. I wanted to lay my weary head on the pillow that Ben bought me for my birthday. A pillow? I hear you ask dear reader. Yes, a pillow. But no ordinary pillow. It's a fully-washable-luxury-microfibre-music-pillow! There's a small speaker inserted inside , which can be connected to a CD or mp3 player. A lovely thoughtful gift.

9.20 p.m.   Rest my head on my luxury music pillow, wriggling my toes to the first track on Danny's CD, *Easy Street*. The song is entitled, *Use Me Up*. I'm all used up, but the rhythm brings life back into my toes, as they happily wiggle under the duvet.

9.24 p.m.   I'm listening to the second track, *Fall At Your Feet*. The tune has my feet rocking from side to side. I sing along ..... *I hope and I pray, and I feel I could fall at your feet..... whooo.*

9.31 p.m.   Track four is a jolly instrumental that chugs along like a happy train. My right knee begins to move to the groove and my eyelashes merrily flutter.

9.33 p.m.   I sing along to *Ease My Blues*.....
You ease my blues away every time.....
You ease my blues away every time.....
This is certainly easing my blues away.

9.36 p.m.	*A Habit I can't Break*, makes my hips move a little from side to side.
9.40 p.m.	I'm resting while I enjoy *She's Got A Hold On Me*, because the following track is one of my favourites, and I know I'll want to bed-dance and sing along to the groove.
9.44 p.m.	Happily singing along in harmony with the chorus..... *Come rain or shine..... whooo* *Come rain or shine..... whooo* I'm bed-dancing from the waist down. Great fun. Hmm, I think I'll request this song when I next see Danny playing at The Pilot.
9.46 p.m.	Decide to listen to *Come Rain Or Shine* again (twice) so I get to know the words and can sing along at Danny's next gig, like a fan at a pop concert.
9.57 p.m.	Listening to *I Got The Blues*, feeling happy and far from blue.
10.01 p.m.	Singing along quietly to myself. *Easy Street* is the song I requested last time I saw Danny play. I can't resist a little bit of bed-dancing, my toes and shoulders wiggle to the rhythm.
10.06 p.m.	Listening to *Easy Street* again, followed by a lovely instrumental.
10.21 p.m.	Danny's arrangement of *Amazing Grace* is amazingly graceful. I feel very relaxed and sleepy.
10.23 p.m.	Dozing to *Not In My Name*. The guitar playing at the end of the song is so incredibly beautiful, I can clearly see in my minds eye, angels dancing on a fast flowing river.
10.29 p.m.	Singing along with the final track, *For You*. The gentle love song, so wonderfully sung, brings tears to my eyes and my voice goes all wobbly.

10.33 p.m.   Blowing nose on Kleenex and smiling, I feel like I've had a *really enjoyable* entertaining night out.

10.36 p.m.   Fall asleep and dream of angels dressed in dazzling white robes, dancing on a fast flowing river of deep-blues.

Tuesday 7th

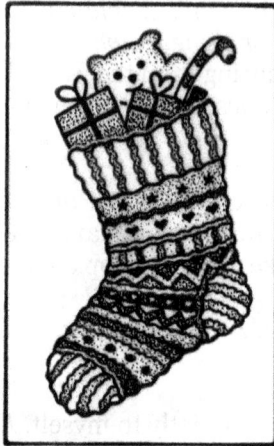

The Christmas stocking in today's Advent calendar window inspired me to wrap a few small gifts for my niece's Christmas stocking. The chocolate bell melted on my tongue like the sound of church bells in the distance, dissolving away into a winter sunset. For a moment I felt poetic, then I sneezed and blew all inspiration into jolly festive kitchen roll. But I *did* feel inspired to find our box of Christmas decorations, and draped some gold tinsel here and there. Then I felt so exhausted, I had to spend the rest of the day in bed reading my Diary 2002 and leafing through today's Christmas catalogues – with the odd cat nap.

My diary entry for May 21st made me giggle, because I'd forgotten I used to enjoy watching home-improvement-type-programmes. Especially the *Big Strong Boys*. Just the title of the programme made me smile.

The team of Big Strong Boys on BBC1 are my new inspiration to get out of bed in the morning. Their charming humour cheers the start of my day; as they transform a huge loft bedroom with clever lighting and animal prints, construct a funky bedroom for a boy, brighten a gloomy kitchen, create a modern look with a fire surround and corner plinth, or give a bedroom a touch of shabby chic.

Today Jake and Gavin remodelled a dining room as a twenties railway carriage, with many features inspired by old fashioned railway stations.

Tonight I felt inspired to create a colourful salad, as I transformed huge crisp lettuce leaves with cubes of bright orange and yellow peppers, dotted artily here and there. I framed funky pasta twirls with slices of evenly spaced cucumber and beetroot, and created a modern look by cutting tomatoes into flower shapes (a dollop of mayonnaise in the middle) sprinkled with sweetcorn nibblets. I gave the pasta (in a crème fraîche dressing with chestnut and wild button mushrooms) a touch of shabby chic, with curled parsley. Then garnished the whole masterpiece with sun kissed chives, freshly picked from my herb garden by my own fair witchy hands. But I forgot the coleslaw.

I laughed out loud when I read my diary entry for 28th May, because I had forgotten how much I used to love watching *Big Brother*, especially the highlights. I even used to get excited about placing a vote for who I wanted to leave or stay in the Big Brother house. Sad but true.

The Eurovision Song Contest was on TV tonight; I felt very fortunate that I missed it, and watched Big Brother instead. Our TV guide says it's the time of year when normally intelligent individuals find their brains turning to mush, as they watch people they don't know, putting all their energies into doing nothing. Well, I have to say, I find it extremely comforting watching other people doing nothing. They eat, sleep, chat a little, visit the bathroom, lie around a lot, cook or clean a little, sometimes feel low and bored, and enjoy the odd bit of entertainment. Like me.

Lands End catalogue sent me their seasonal collection of Pima polos, Fair Isle roll necks, Argyle cardigans, and fleecy cowl neck sweaters. All in glorious shades of vivid plum, iris, spice brown, maplewood, arctic grey, and velvet plum. Woods Supplements sent their collection of best sellers: echinacea, evening primrose oil, ginger extract, kelp extract, grapeseed extract, bilberry extract.......

BBC Audio Books sent a catalogue of their seasonal collection of classic fiction, adventure and comedy; including *The Adventure of the Christmas pudding* by Agatha Christie, *I'm sorry I haven't a Christmas clue*, and *Village Christmas* by Miss Read. I decided to order a book to add to my collection (a Christmas gift to myself) but the thought of addressing an envelope, filling in a form, writing out a cheque, and popping it all in the envelope, made me feel so tired I nodded off to sleep. I dreamt my book, *Love & Best Witches*, was made into an audio book and became a seasonal best seller.

When I awoke smiling late afternoon, I listened to a CD of a BBC comedy TV series from the seventies, *Morecambe and Wise*. There was a joke I thought Ben would like to tell at his Avocado Pair gig that evening.

ME: I was listening to Morecambe and Wise today.

BEN: That's nice dear.

ME: I'd forgotten how hilarious they were!

BEN: Yeah, I remember watching the shows.

ME: Mmm me too, and there was a joke I thought you'd like to tell at your gig tonight.

BEN: Yeah?

ME: It wasn't the apple that caused all the trouble in the Garden of Eden, it was the pair on the ground.

BEN: Hahaha, great!

ME: I'd like to visit the Eden project in the West Country next summer, I'll have a wheelchair by then.

BEN: Good idea.

ME: You will be able to push me around as much as you like!

BEN: Wonderful idea, and maybe we could look for homes on the Cornish coast.

ME: Fabulous idea, we could probably afford half a beach hut. Or the steps leading up to it.

Wednesday 8th

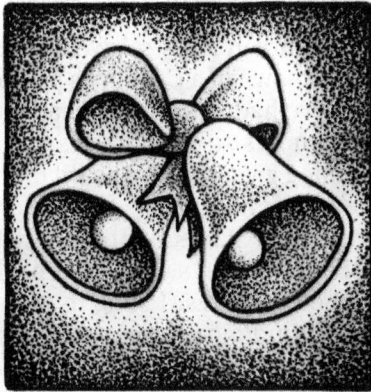

      I spent the night in the Garden of Eden with Ben, enjoying an avocado pear picnic. He tempted me with a strawberry cupcake, hanging from a strawberry cupcake tree. I couldn't resist the pink delight, and after one bite I woke up craving something strawberry flavoured. I fancied strawberry jam on toast, but we didn't have any strawberry jam, so I had banana on toast instead. That was nice and sweet, and would give me some slow burning energy to start writing Christmas cards. The chocolate Christmas pudding in today's Advent window was nice and sweet too, and gave me a little instant energy to reply to Ben's text message.

9.09 a.m.   THINK I-VE LEFT MY SQUIDS FROM LAST NITE-S GIG IN MY
             TROUSERS - CAN U CHECK ?

9.12 a.m.   YES U DID - CAN U GET FRESH PIZZA ON WAY HOME - TOO
             TIRED TO COOK DINS TONITE ?

9.15 a.m.   WILL DO X

9.16 a.m.   OH - CAN U GET STRAWBERRY JAM TOO - SUGAR FREE IF
             POSS

9.17 a.m.   OK

9.18 A.M.   THANX X

The little picture in today's Advent window was two golden
bells, tied with a red satin bow, on a Cadbury's purple background. They
made me grin because I've had bells in my head for days. Not just my
tinnitus; jingle bells. Ben has started practising Christmas songs to
play at his Tuesday evening gigs, and I've heard the tune to *Jingle Bells*,
over and over *and over* again.

Late afternoon I started writing Christmas cards, I chose
six with a picture of Santa on his sleigh. When I had written all the
cards and addressed the envelopes, I sang to myself with a *job-well-
done* smile on my face, *'Jingle bells, jingle bells, jingle all the way'*.
Then I curled up with my cats to read more of my Diary 2002.

My diary entry for 26th May was interesting, because it
was a detailed account of a visit to our local garden centre (I can't
believe how long I stayed on my feet). Britain would soon be celebrating
the Queen's Golden Jubilee, so the names of the plants filling the
entrance amused me: Golden Tiara, Campanula Elizabeth, and Rose
Golden Jubilee, to name a few.

Ben and I leisurely wandered around admiring shrubs,
fuchsias, hydrangeas, wild flowers and herbs. I liked the names of some
of the wild flowers: Corncockle, Bell flower, Bird's foot Trefoil and
Maiden Pink. I could almost *see* the fairies dancing among the leaves.
I gazed in wonder at the little alpine rock gardens, and beautiful roses
with lovely names like, Dawn Chorus and New Dawn. Then, after a

visit to the water feature and garden ornament section, I started to wilt, like the plants that needed watering.

The stripy sun loungers looked extremely inviting for a very tired person. I desperately needed to sit down for a while. I pretended to be terribly interested in the marvellous picnic baskets, as I sat trying out the magnificently made hard wood garden bench. It was such a beautiful bench, I had to admire it for a while. Quite a long while. Ben sat beside me, and we commented on the lovely colour of the wood. And what a truly wonderful smooth finish. I commented that Jake and Gavin would love it. Then of course Ben wanted to know who Jake and Gavin were; so naturally we had to sit for a while longer, as I told him all about the Big Strong Boys. Then we pretended to admire the bench again, agreeing that it would look perfect in our garden, facing west, so we could sit and watch the sun set in our golden jubilee years.

Two sweet, cheerful old ladies wearing flowery dresses, were trying out the patio chairs. They giggled, probably needing a rest like me. But it wasn't just me and the old ladies who were tired. A small boy, about five years old, sat on a blue plastic cool box wearing a Bob the Builder cap, slumped in a weary way like a tired builder in his lunch hour. His mother and grandmother were busy admiring garden lanterns with much enthusiasm. He couldn't see what all the fuss was about, as he sighed a big man sigh. I could see him in twenty years time on a building site, sitting on a pile of bricks with his sausage sandwiches in his lunch hour. He would sigh a big man sigh, waiting for the week to end, so he could take the wife and mother~in~law to the garden centre to buy lanterns; he couldn't see the point.

On our way out of the garden centre I noticed a lonely, thirsty looking tomato plant in a pot. All by himself. The pot had fallen on it's side, and as I sat it upright, I noticed his name was Big Boy ~ a vigorous tomato with very large tasty fruits.

Back home, feet up, Big Boy tomato plant sitting happily with his thirst quenched (in our kitchen) I read the instructions on how to care for him. He needed to be grown in a greenhouse. We haven't got a greenhouse. I decided to sit him in a sunny sheltered spot and keep my green witchy fingers crossed.

7.46 p.m.   Ben was working on the chords to another Christmas song, *Winter Wonderland* .... B... F#... F#7... C#M... F#... E... C#M9...

7.50 p.m.   I started to sing along, but felt frustrated that I didn't know many of the words.

ME: Would you mind printing out the words to the songs you're practising, so I can sing along?

BEN: Certainly dear.

Thursday 9th

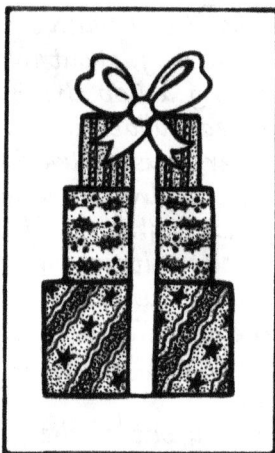

8.25 a.m.   Switched the kettle on for my morning cuppa, and sang to the cats.

Sleigh bells ring, are you listening

In the lane, snow is glistening
A beautiful sight we're happy tonight
Walking in a winter wonderland

9.30 a.m.   Filled the bird table and sang to the birds.

Gone away is the bluebird
Here to stay is a new bird
He sings a love song, as we go along
Walking in a winter wonderland

9.45 a.m.   Noticed the snowman in the car park had completely melted away. I sang to the car park.

In the meadow we can build a snowman
Then pretend that he is Parson Brown
He'll say: Are you married? We'll say: No man
But you can do the job when you're in town

10.00 a.m.   Sang to myself as I did the washing-up.

Later on we'll conspire
As we dream by the fire
To face unafraid, the plans that we made
Walking in a winter wonderland

11.40 a.m.   Opened the morning post. Just one Christmas card; a winter wonderland of trees sparkling in the snow, with a sprinkling of green glitter here and there. That's one I will keep for my collection.

11.43 a.m.   Opened my Advent calendar window. The picture was a pile of Christmas gifts tied with a bow, and the chocolate snowflake melted on my tongue like my heart, when Cleopatra gave my nose a good wash first thing this morning.

12.30 p.m.   Inspired by the picture in my calendar window, I wrapped three Christmas gifts then wrote three Christmas cards.

4.00 p.m.   As I lay in the bath under mountains of white froth, like the lawn under a lumpy blanket of snow, I sang to the bubbles.

When it snows, ain't it thrilling
Though your nose gets a chilling
We'll frolic and play, the Eskimo way
Walking in a winter wonderland

5.00 p.m.   I lay on the sofa, under a lumpy blanket of cats, and read a few more entries in my Diary 2002.

June 3rd

An entertaining evening. I watched the extended Jubilee episode of Coronation Street, followed by Big Brother, which is getting exciting with more nominations. Alex is very chatty. Kate fancies Spencer. Sunita wants to leave. Jade waxed Alison's braids. Lynn has left and Sandy is looking very miserable. My Big Boy tomato plant is looking happy, bigger and stronger, with his leaves outstretched. I talk to him, telling him the latest news in the Big Brother house.

June 8th

The Big Strong Boys created a Mediterranean hallway in a semi in Walford today. I loved all the bright blues, sunny yellows and greens. It's been chilly and rainy lately, so I've brought my Big Boy indoors and sat him in the kitchen window. He's pretending he's in a greenhouse. I don't need to tell him the latest goings on in the Big Brother house, I just turn the TV up a little. I'm sure he's started to lean ever so slightly towards the direction of the TV, a leaf to his ear.

June 14th

The housemates in the Big Brother house got a telling off today, they looked like naughty school children. And there was a bit of excitement when Sandy tried to escape from the house, climbing onto the roof. I told Big Boy I wasn't surprised about this, and I was sad Alison had left the house.

His leaves drooped a little. But when I re~potted him in his new bigger pot, gave him a drink and sat him outside in the hot sunshine, he soon brightened up.

June 18th
Jake and Gavin transformed a blue boy's room into a Gothic castle today. They built a wooden castle wall, with turrets and a drawbridge round the bunk beds. They made colourful shields and flags too. Fabulous. Big Boy is looking fabulous as well; tall green and handsome, almost fifteen inches in height now. I brought him indoors during a storm today, and gently shook the raindrops from his leaves. I sat him in the nice warm sitting room to recover from the scary thunder and lightening, and we watched Big Brother together. Today Adele had her first shower in seven days. I know how she feels ~ absolutely fabulous.

June 23rd
Big Brother made me feel sad today because I was feeling sorry for Kate. She was missing Spencer so much, she slept in his bed. I like Kate. Jonny was feeling low because he regretted nominating Spencer for eviction. And I'm still missing Alison. When I told all this to Big Boy, his leaves drooped a lot, or maybe it was the big fat raindrops resting on his leaves. When I mentioned Alex had won <u>another</u> task, then gave his branches a little shake, he perked~up straight away.

June 30th
The Big Strong Boys were in Spain today, I could <u>almost</u> <u>feel</u> the heat glowing out of the TV screen, and the sky was <u>so</u> <u>blue</u>. Jake and Gavin were busy working on a plain, cold looking white bedroom in a villa, making it cosy and comfortable. They made a new bed, arched mirror and drawers. There was lots of terracotta paintwork, lots of green plants, and drapes with a Roman feel. Big Boy is enjoying the warmth of my kitchen again because it's cold and windy outside. He's looking

strong and confident, twenty inches tall now; and I expect he'd like to be with the Big Strong Boys at the moment, soaking up Spanish sunbeams. But we enjoyed the psychological analysis of the Big Brother housemates; soon they will all be evicted, but one.

Friday 10th

> *The moon on the breast of new~fallen snow*
> *Gave the lustre of mid~day to objects below,*
> *When, what to my wondering eyes should appear,*
> *But a miniature sleigh, and eight tiny reindeer.*

From a poem called 'Night Before Christmas'
By Major Henry Livingstone Jr.

Two more Christmas cards arrived with the post today. The first one I opened had a picture of Santa on his sleigh, with an extract from a poem. The second one showed a tiny fairy dressing a Christmas tree, from my aunt and uncle in Yorkshire. With their card was another charming little card with a photo of a tulip on the front, written by their eight year old grand daughter, Elsa. Inside the card was a message to her fairy friend, Lucey (Elsa's spelling).

Elsa loves to climb a cedar tree in their garden, where she hides a card to Lucey. When she goes home after a visit; my aunt retrieves the letter, then writes a reply (from Lucey) which she leaves among the flowers in her porch for Elsa to find on her next visit. How magical!

A smiling Santa waved at me when I opened my Advent calendar window; the present shaped chocolate melting in my mouth, like my heart going all soft, when I read letters written to Santa in Weekly Wife by little children.

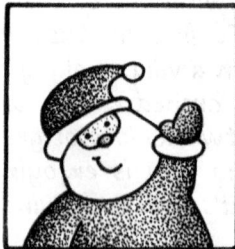

Dear Santa
I've been a really good big sister
to my new baby sister, Emily.
Please bring me a Barbie Glam
Vacation House. We will leave you
a mince pie and some carrots
for your reindeer. And we'll
leave you a cup with a teabag
in so you can make yourself a
cup of tea. Thank you Santa.

Chloe, aged 6

Dear Santa
Because I have been helping
Mummy, Daddy and my big brother
Joshua, Mummy said I can ask you
for a parachute and metal detector
so I can look for treasure like the
Power Rangers. Please don't forget
me or Joshua as we are not at the
same house as last year. Thank you.

Samuel, aged 5

Dear Santa
I've just started school and because
I've been a good girl I'd really like
some sparkly shoes. I'd also like
some Hello Kitty stickers and a
toy baby, so I can look after her
like Mummy looks after my little
sister, Emma.

Matilda, aged 4

I wrapped a few bottles of Santa's Wobble beer; putting them in a jiffy bag first, so they would be easier to wrap and wouldn't clank in Santa's sack when he climbed down the chimney. Then I wrote three Christmas letters; enclosing them in cards with a smiling Santa on the front, riding on a sleigh with piles of presents. By the end of the day I felt like I'd done a good days work. I lay on the sofa, closed my eyes, and thought about writing a letter to Santa. I would tell him I'd been a good girl this year; taking my supplements and pacing myself as much as possible, so could I have some sparkly shoes (with black sequins, from ACE catalogue) and sparkly bath goodies from Lush. Then I would put, P.S. I've left brandy and mince pies for you, and some carrots for your reindeer.

Or maybe I'd send him the text message Jayne sent me the other day, for a laugh.

HI SANTA – FOR 2011 – ALL I WANT IS A FAT BANK ACCOUNT AND A SKINNY BODY – LETS TRY NOT TO MIX UP THE TWO – LIKE LAST YEAR – OK ?

Saturday 11th

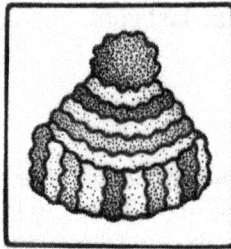

9.45 a.m.   There was a woolly bobble hat in today's calendar window, and the chocolate Christmas pudding melted on my tongue like a snowflake on a bobble hat, worn on a hot head.

11. 45 a.m.   Hurrah! Hurrah! *Hurrah! Hurrrrraaaaahhhhh!!!!!!!!!!!*
My copy of InterAction magazine arrived from A.F.M.E. I turned straight to page 28, and there it was, m*y very own DOUBLE PAGE SPREAD.* It looked wonderful. I felt like a model who had finally achieved success, with her photo

on the cover of Vogue magazine, except this was *much more exciting!*

11.50 a.m.   I curled up with my cats on the sofa, browsing through InterAction. I read Stacy Heart's page first, because it always makes me laugh, and a witch needs a good cackle at least once a week.

2.25 p.m.   I wanted to dress up, and go out to a country pub for a meal to celebrate my wonderful double-page spread. I day dreamt of having a book launch party, inviting my family and friends, with Robbie Williams for entertainment. But I knew I had to conserve my energy for Christmas preparations, and visiting my family on Christmas day. And I *had* told Santa I was being a good girl. *So* I put a bottle of Merlot on the shopping list, and Ben said he'd cook a special vege curry.

4.00 p.m.   Cosy and warm under a blanket of tabby cats, I read entries for July in my Diary 2002.

July 4th

The Big Strong Boys were looking rather subdued today, now that they were back in rainy England, after their time in sunny Spain. They sawed and sanded oak beams, and created atmospheric lighting (with a touch of Spanish warmth) in a dismal, grey looking living room. Big Boy looked very droopy, so I gently shook the raindrops from his leaves, and gave him some plant food. I told him all about the latest nominations in the Big Brother house, and he started to look very uplifted.

July 10th

It's day 47 in the Big Brother house, and the housemates are sleeping off their hangovers after last night's party. It's day 16 for my Big Boy in his new home with his new housemates, Ben, the cats and me. Although I'm not keeping him in a greenhouse, he seems happy enough in his sheltered corner, and the weather is hot today. Jake and Gavin were big strong sunny boys today, as they worked on a plain large lounge. They made a storage place in a bay window, created big chunky units, waxed and buffed the floor, and added a simple fireplace with a modern mirror. Some of the woodwork was given a distressed look. I only need to look in the bathroom mirror first thing in the morning, to get a distressed look!

July 15th

Big Boy is flourishing. He's 28 inches tall now, with three little yellow flowers. I re~plotted him and he enjoyed a lovely long drink. The housemates in the Big Brother house enjoyed a croquet set, as a reward for cleaning the pool. The Big Strong Boys decorated two bedrooms for two little boys, Max and Archie. Lots of bold primary colours, a toy storage box, drums and trumpets painted on the walls, and a wooden hobby horse. Lucky Max and Archie, I'd love a room just like that.

July 20th

Before my morning de~caf tea, I gave Big Boy his morning drink and told him the latest news from the Big Brother house. There's only four housemates left now (Kate, Jade, Alex and Jonny) and they were awarded a beach party after last night's task. I don't want any of them to leave, I like them all. I mentioned this to my Big Boy and he nodded in agreement, or maybe it was the gentle summer breeze moving his leaves. Jake and Gavin gave a country house a seaside look today. I fancy a trip to the seaside. Hastings. Or maybe Whitstable.

July 26th

It's the hottest July since 1989. I can well believe it. The Big Strong Boys were busy knocking down a kitchen wall for today's theme, a Mexican desert. Lots of MDF sawing, sawdust, terracotta, painted wooden chilli peppers, a spice rack, and lots of bright green, red and yellow paintwork. Lovely. My Big Boy looks colourful too, he has six yellow flowers now, and he's a big strong boy, at thirty eight inches tall. Tonight was the last night of the evictions in the Big Brother house. I rang Channel 4 on

09011 15 4410 to vote for Kate to win. And she won ~ hurrah! That would most probably be my big excitement for 2002. Although I'm looking forward to my Big Boy bearing fruit.

8. 00 p.m.   After dinner we drank wine and sang along to Ben's guitar, as he rehearsed a Christmas tune for his next gig.

ME: *Oh, the weather outside is frightful,*
But the snow is so delightful,
And since we've no place to go,

BEN: *Let it snow! Let it snow! Let it snow!*

ME: *It doesn't show signs of stopping,*
And I've bought some corn for popping,
The lights are turned down low,

BEN: *Let it snow! Let it snow! Let it snow!*

8.15 p.m.   *Cheers A.F.M.E. !*

Sunday 12th

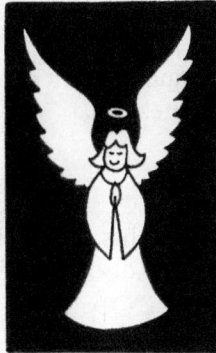

9.16 a.m.   After filling the bird table and hanging bird feeders, I stood silently gazing up at the sycamore trees. Several grey collared doves perched on the branches, bobbing in the breeze. They brought to mind Christmas tree decorations, perfectly placed, pretty as a picture. I counted them, there were twelve. So naturally I burst into song, *'On the twelfth day of Christmas my true love sent to me, doves in a sycamore tree.'*

9.20 a.m.   I plodded indoors and watched the doves from the warmth of my kitchen. They flew down onto the bird table, fence and feeders, like small children descending on their presents under the tree, early Christmas morning. I decided to call them my twelve doves of Christmas.

9.25 a.m.   As I went to open my Advent calendar window, I realised it was the twelfth. The window opened to reveal an angel in white, on a Cadbury's purple background. The chocolate robin melted, like my heart when I read about the Christmas Angel project in InterAction.

10.51 a.m.   When I read some facts about chocolate in Weekly Wife, I knew Ben would be *most* interested.

ME: Ounce for ounce, dark chocolate has seventeen times the antioxidant power of oranges.

BEN: That's interesting dear.

ME: *Yes!* And good quality dark chocolate is a source of iron, copper and magnesium.

BEN: Marvellous.

ME: Cocoa butter contains oleic acid, a healthy cholesterol-lowering fat, that is also found in avocados.

BEN: Fascinating.

ME: You know that song about the twelve days of Christmas?

BEN: Yeah. Don't tell me, there's a new version where the true love sends twelve boxes of chocolates.

ME: *No dear*, but you've inspired me to write a chocolaty festive song! That will be something exciting to do tomorrow. I've been singing the twelve days of Christmas song today, and I can remember all the words except one bit. Do you know what the true love sends on the ninth day of Christmas?

BEN: Erm, eleven pipers piping, ten drummers drumming...... how about nine lead guitarists ?

3.15 p.m.   Ben sent me a text message as he was about to leave his nephew Alex's house:

POPPIN INTO SAINS-B ON WAY HOME - ANYTHIN U-D LIKE?

3. 16 p.m.   I replied:

MMM, YES - ON THE TWELFTH DAY OF DECEMBER YOU BOUGHT IN SAINSBURY - 12 BARS OF CHOCOLATE - AND A PARTRIDGE IN A PEAR TREE

3.17 p.m.   Ben replied:

WOT R U LIKE ?

3.18 p.m.   I DUNNO WOT I'M LIKE, BUT I DO KNOW A BAR OF PLAIN CHOC WUD BE DIVINE - THANX X

Monday 13th

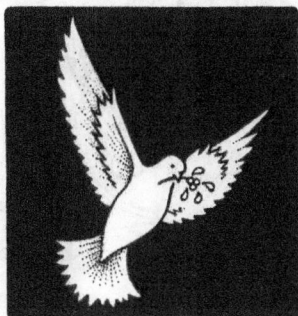

A white dove in flight (on a Cadbury's purple background) greeted me when I opened today's window. The chocolate holly melting on my tongue, like my heart melted when I opened today's Christmas card; a fluffy white kitten, wearing a red Santa hat. I wanted to hold a tiny fluffy white kitten in my arms. I wanted to see millions of white fluffy snowflakes falling from the sky. Instead of raindrops on roses, I wanted to see snowflakes on roses and whiskers on kittens. There's nothing like a few of your favourite things to cheer you up.

My Monday morning misty blues lifted when I noticed Bobby robin bobbing along on our garden fence. As I admired his bright orangy-red breast, I thought about my breasts; it was about time I booked a cancer check. As I gazed at Bobby's fine feathers, I plucked up the courage to pick up the phone and make an appointment.

The hospital in Tunbridge Wells could see me on Friday afternoon, 1.00 p.m. 8th January. Great. That would give me time to recover from visiting my family on Christmas day. I thought about writing to Santa, telling him I'd been a good girl and booked for a test, so could I have the beautiful bra and briefs set I've seen in La Redoute catalogue. Very feminine. Champagne or rosewood embroidered tulle, combining comfort and softness. If they haven't got my size, I also like the raspberry pink nightshirt with Hello Kitty motif.

Prestige Cellars sent me a posh looking letter with their catalogue. The coat of arms (with a goblet and barrel) made me smile.

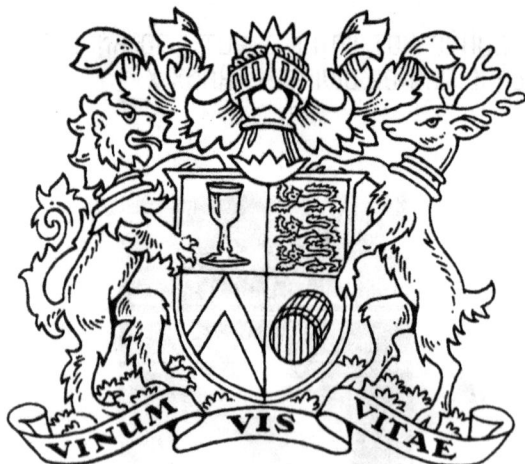

Their catalogue was amusing to read too .... *gifts perfect for grumpy old men everywhere. Don't delay and miss the sleigh .... Wine and food presents that even Scrooge can afford and Santa would be proud to deliver .... Gifts to bring a heart-warming glow to givers and receivers, even those hard to please people .... Tasty gifts for Hot Chocoholics .... 'Old Git' gift sets (ale or wine).*

2. 21 p.m.   The bubbles in my bath inspired me to make up a chocolaty festive song. I sang softly to my breasts, hidden under a duvet of bubbles. They needed cheering up because they don't want to go for a cancer check, even though I've told them it's for their own good.........*'On the first day of Christmas my true love sent to me a partridge in a pear tree...........On the second day of Christmas my true love sent to me, two boxes of Maltesers and a partridge in a pear tree...........On the third day of Christmas my true love sent to me.........three boxes of Matchmakers, three different flavours, orange,mint and coffee.........'*

2. 21 p.m.   Started having chocolate cravings (I so love a nice cold crispy Matchmaker, especially mint flavour) so I had to stop, and sing about Rudolf the red nosed reindeer.

Tuesday 14th

9. 15 a.m.   I found today's window on Santa's reindeer's bum. The little picture was a Christmas cake, decorated with a robin, snowman, and a Christmas tree. The chocolate Santa melted in my mouth like snowflakes on a warm reindeer's bum.

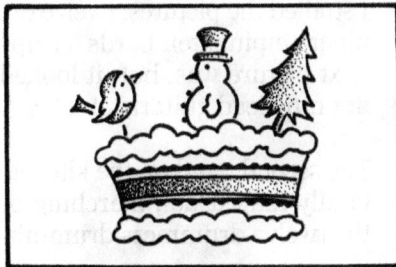

9.30 a.m.   I sat my weary bum on the kitchen stool to watch the birds feed, and gaze sleepily at the bare sycamore tree branches, dark against a pale blue sky. I admired the shapes of light between the branches. Then as I turned my head away from the wintry scene (to put the kettle on) I blinked, and a beautiful intricate pattern of the tree branches appeared on the white kettle (white branches on a grey background). I blinked again and the pattern appeared on the white kitchen roll, then on the white electric can opener. That was fun.

10.30 a.m.   I lay in the bath dreaming of a white Christmas, under snowy-white clouds, enjoying the sound of tiny bubbles popping all around me. I breathed in the sweet scent of pine, emanating from Christmas-tree-green tea-lights at the tap end of the bath. Ben bought them for me at the weekend, from Sainsbury's. I was surprised when he gave them to me, I had never seen Christmas-tree-green tea-lights before. Another fun moment.

10.40 a.m.   Still in the bath, I gazed at two shampoo bottles sitting in the bathroom window. As bright winter-afternoon-white shone through the frosted pane, the bottles appeared to glow. One, a golden yellow, the other a vibrant bluey-green. After a while I averted my gaze to the frosted window pane. I blinked. Two fuzzy bottle shapes appeared. The yellow bottle was now lilac, the bluey-green, now pink. *Another fun moment.*

11.30 a.m.   Today's Christmas card was the twelve days of Christmas. I studied the pictures: twelve drummers drumming, eleven pipers piping, ten Lords a leaping. I wasn't sure what the next picture was, but it looked like nine ladies dancing, not nine lead guitarists!

11.32 a.m.   The second hand on the kitchen clock seemed to tick more loudly than usual, marching on towards Christmas, like the twelve drummers drumming.

11.35 a.m.   My newsletter arrived from the Kent and Sussex ME/CFS Society. I like their newsletter because there's *always* something I find really interesting or helpful. I leafed through until I found the advert for my witchy book. As soon as I spotted it I felt a bubble of excitement, like the Christmas morning when I was six, and I *knew* the strange, almost coffin shaped box, would be a tiny acoustic guitar.

5.00 p.m.   After wrapping a few presents and writing some cards, I curled up with the furry children to read more of my Diary 2002.

August 3rd

My Big Boy tomato plant has one pale green tomato, the size of a large marble, and pumpkin shaped. He enjoyed a refreshing light summer shower today, in between sunny spells. I noticed tiny spiders have made their homes, their intricate delicate webs, across his upper leaves. A witch enjoys a lovely pumpkin shaped tomato, spider webs and sunny spells.

August 10th

Storms woke me up during the night. They sounded like God rolling huge stone boulders down his stairway to heaven. I checked on my Big Boy first thing. His leaves were droopy and sleepy with morning raindrops, so I gave his branches a little shake. He woke up and sparkled in the morning sun. I was pleased to see his one tomato was still thriving. The Big Strong Boys transformed a bedroom for two children, Celeste and Nathan; sky blue walls with fluffy white clouds, a kite mobile, hot air balloon mirror, and cloud shaped picture frames. Lovely. I miss Big Brother. Watched the film Big, <u>so</u> love Tom Hanks.

August 14th

Hurrah! Big Boy has sprouted another green tomato! Now I'm broody for more green babies. Jake and

Gavin turned an attic into a multi~functional room: a play room and a guest bedroom. Laminate floor, jazzed~up doors, lanterns, storage for toys, pale blue and purple paintwork. It was unusual stripy paintwork ~ very effective.

August 19th

Ben bought fresh Scottish strawberries. I've never had <u>Scottish</u> strawberries! They were <u>most</u> delicious, very juicy and beautifully shaped. Must be the wonderful Highland air. I hoped my Big Boy would produce lots of beautifully pumpkin shaped, juicy red fruits. I had a feeling he would. He has more flowers and six baby green tomatoes now, various sizes. I've been sitting in the sun telling him about the Big Strong Boys' latest transformations, and I've grown more freckles, various sizes.

August 24th

Jake and Gavin looked very cheerful to be back in sunny Spain. Today they converted a guest bedroom into a country cottage for a British couple. Big Boy looked disappointed with the chilly and cloudy British weather, but his green babies are still growing. One is almost the size of a tennis ball.

6.15 p.m.   I showed Ben the advert for my book in the Kent and Sussex M.E./CFS newsletter.

ME: Looks great doesn't it!

BEN: Yeah!

ME: I'm glad you've got a gig tonight, I'm exhausted.

BEN: That's no wonder, looks like you've been busy.

ME: I have. I've wrapped pressies, written cards and letters, and parcelled them up. Can you post them on Saturday please?

BEN: Yep.

ME: Thanks (big yawn).

Wednesday 15th

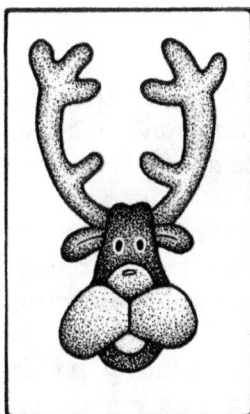

      A jolly reindeer greeted me in today's Advent window. The chocolate Christmas tree melted on my tongue, like my heart melted when I saw a photo of Blue in Weekly Wife; the first reindeer calf to be born in Britain since the ice age. He was born recently at the Trevarno Estate, Helston in Cornwall. They have several reindeer there: Dancer, Rudolf, Prancer, Dasher, Vixen, Donna, Blitzen, Cupid, Glider and Comet. I would love to see them one day; I collect cuddly toy reindeer and have *always* wanted to see a *real* one.

2. 35 p.m.   I leafed through September's entries in my Diary 2002.

September 8th

      My Gardener's Calendar 2002, says September is the first of the autumn months, and whilst there is still much to enjoy in the garden, it is now time to start planning for next year. Well, I plan to do as little as possible, now and next year. Sit and talk to the trees and the birds. Pass the time with ladybirds and caterpillars. Chat about the weather and rising cost of peanuts with the squirrels. Water and care for another tomato plant and my herbs. A witch must have her herbs. I watered my Big Boy, his branches weighed down with big fat green tomatoes. I miss the Big Strong Boys, their D.I.Y. programme is over. Watched Big Business instead, with Bette Middler and Lily Tomlin. Felt better.

September 13th

It's Friday 13th, unlucky for some. But lucky for me, because my Big Boy now has thirteen healthy looking green baby fruits. I told him I've started watching Garden Invaders. Today they were in a huge garden on the Isle of Wight, where Kim Wilde styled a fish pond and tidied a vegetable patch. I've started watching House Invaders too. Today they were in Halifax, transforming a kitchen hell into a cook's heaven with lots of blues and silver. They also turned a boring bedroom into an exciting paradise, with lots of lilacs and smoky greens. That was my colourful excitement for the week.

September 22nd

I sipped my morning cuppa of peppermint tea in the garden, enjoying the autumn sunshine warming my face, and a gentle autumn breeze lifting my hair. I admired Big Boy's largest firm fruit, now sporting pale orange and green stripes. I told him about Janice and Fiz, who were sewing stripy underwear at Underworld in Coronation Street. He didn't seem interested, I think he misses hearing about Jake and Gavin. In House Invaders today, the colourful stripes they painted in a bedroom were not my cup of tea. Neither was the lighting in a vegetable patch in Garden Invaders. Both programmes were not a patch on the Big Strong Boys.

September 25th

It was a bright and beautiful autumn day, although the wind was very chilly. The sun shone on Big Boy's huge orangy~red tomato, and twelve smaller green fruits of various sizes. *I hoped, despite the cold weather, all his tomatoes would turn from green to orange, then red; as the autumn leaves turn from green to orange, and red. Nature's traffic lights telling us to slow down for the winter and rest.*

7.22 p.m.   I mentioned the article about the Trevarno Estate to Ben, and he found their website on his computer. There were many photos of all the reindeer, and I swooned, in a reindeer loving way.

ME: Ooh, can we visit there one day, when I'm well enough to travel?

BEN: Yeah, of course!

ME: Oh, goody. Did you know Santa's reindeer must have been female because male reindeer lose their antlers in winter.

BEN: No dear.

ME: Reindeer are excellent swimmers and a day old reindeer is capable of outrunning a man!

BEN: That's interesting dear.

*   *   *   *   *   *   *

8.16 p.m.   Ben rehearsed another Christmas song, and we sang along.

ME: *Rudolf the red~nosed reindeer, had a very shiny nose.*

BEN: *And if you ever saw him, you would even say it glows.*

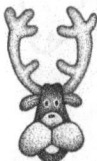

Thursday 16ᵗʰ

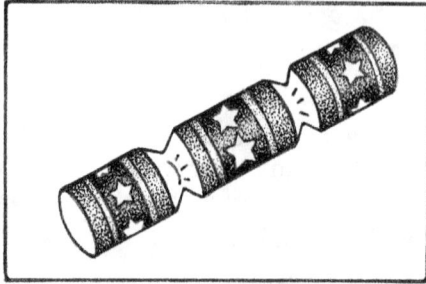

Four Christmas cards arrived with the post today. A tabby kitten curled up asleep in a Santa hat, meerkats wearing Santa hats, and two winter wonderland scenes, sunlight sparkling magically on the snow. I wished for more snow. When I had fed the wildlife earlier, an icy-cold breeze had whispered in my ear of snowflakes, and my sensitive witchy nose could smell approaching snow clouds. The leaves on the privet hedge shivered.

I turned the heating up. My cats purred with approval. I smiled, then opened today's Advent calendar window, to find a cracker. The chocolate present melted warmly in my mouth, like my heart when I opened the kitten-in-a-Santa-hat card. It was from my niece Louise, and she had drawn a picture of two reindeer inside. One had a big red nose, and both had beautiful TV aerial shaped antlers. I hoped she would like the card I sent her just as much; a mother polar bear cuddling her baby bear.

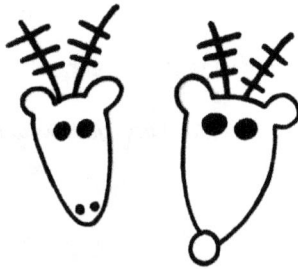

3.23 p.m.   I browsed through October's entries in in my Diary 2002.

October 3rd

Tonight we enjoyed my Big Boy's first huge, ripe pumpkin shaped tomato. Half each, with vege~sausages, baked beans, and a baked potato. Ben agreed, it tasted deliciously fresh and home grown with no artificial anythings. Coronation Street went down well too. Lovesick Sunita spilled the beans to Dev about Geena and Joe's plot to pull the wool over his eyes, and he decided to see just how far the sulky barmaid was prepared to go, in order to keep up the charade.

October 16th

Mother Nature must have enjoyed baked beans, there were very strong winds last night. I checked on Big Boy first thing this morning, and noticed one orangy~red tomato lay on the ground. I picked it up to take safely indoors. The rest of his fruits were still firmly attached to their branches; two were orangy~red, two greeny~orange, and seven pale limey~green. The garden Invaders were quite good today, they transformed a neglected back garden into a woodland haven. The House Invaders were good too, they gave a bedroom a Moroccan look. Very stylish. Although I think the Big Strong Boys would have done a much better job.

October 25th

Big Boy needed cheering up after last night's wind and rain. He had one broken branch and there were two green tomatoes lying on the ground. I wished we had a greenhouse, as I picked up the forlorn fruits, then gently shook the rain from his leaves and told him about yesterday's Garden Invaders.

ME: They featured a natural~style pond, it was lovely and became the focal point of the garden. Kim

Wilde was good, I like her, she gave lots of advice on aquatic plants.

BIG BOY: Do you have a pond? (tomato language).

ME: No, but I will have one day.

BIG BOY: What are you like (tomato language).

ME: I notice you have two more beautiful ripe fruits, may I pick them?

BIG BOY: Go ahead, I've grown them especially for you (tomato language).

ME: Oh, wonderful, a tomato has never said that to me before! Would you like me to give your stem another little shake, get rid of more raindrops?

BIG BOY: Oh, yes....... ah, that's better (tomato language).

October 31ˢᵗ

This morning I wished Big Boy a happy Halloween, as I picked two more of his ripened fruits. And he did look happier, as if two little weights had been lifted from his shoulders. The sun shone brightly. I felt uplifted too, as I told him about the Harry Potter special I had seen; a behind the scenes of the upcoming film, Chamber of Secrets. I'm so looking forward to it, having read J.K. Rowling's wonderful book.

This afternoon, I noticed two little school girls galloping down our street on toy broomsticks at going~home~time. They joyfully screamed and cackled. A tiny boy watched them, completely spellbound, from his pushchair.

Tonight I cut the eyes, nose, and mouth (Halloween pumpkin style) out of Big Boy's pumpkin shaped tomatoes. We relished them with vege spicy bean burgers, sweetcorn, and monster mash (instant mash , made black with food colouring).

6.24 p.m. Louise sent me a text message:

YOUR CARD IS REALLY SWEET – THANKS X

6.25 p.m. I replied:

LOVED YOUR KITTEN CARD TOO – CAN-T WAIT TO GIVE YOU YOUR XMAS PREZZIE – IT-S SO YOU – BEST XMAS WITCHES WITH TINSLE ON THEIR BROOMSTICKS X

6. 30 p.m. Louise replied:

AHHH, REALLY? - SOUNDS GREAT – CAN-T WAIT TO SEE YOU X

6.46 p.m. Jayne sent me a text message:

HEY WITCHY FRIEND – I-VE SENT U THE REVIEW OF YOR BOOK ON MY SITE – HAV U SEEN THE NEW HARRY POTTER MOVIE ?

7.35 p.m. Ben showed me Jayne's review on his computer. I picked up my mobile as soon as I had read it, and texted her:

OOOH, WOT A LUVLI REVIEW – THANX SO MUCH FOR ALL YOR THORT AND EFFORT – VERY MUCH APPRECIATED – BEN SAW THE HARRY P MOVIE – I-M WAITING TO SEE IT ON DVD – BEST WITCHES XVX

9.15 p.m. I stared out of the kitchen window and thought I may be *seeing* things. Did the lawn look a little white in places?

9.16 p.m. I opened the front door, and was delighted to see I had not been imagining things. The cars parked in our street were covered in a thin layer of snow; the curved bonnets, like the top of a Victoria sponge cake, sprinkled with a generous amount of icing sugar.

Friday 17th

My morning was very pleasant. I sat in the warmth of our cosy kitchen, watching huge fluffy white snowflakes silently fall from the cold grey skies, transforming the garden into a delightful snow globe. My boiling eggs were softly bubbling. The toast was happily toasting, filling the room with a delicious comforting aroma. Toasty warm cats were purring and grooming. A Kit-Kat mug of peppermint tea was steaming peppermintly. My tired heart smiled.

I leafed through the November entries in my Diary 2002; I was keen to see how my Big Boy tomato plant had fared in the cold weather. November 1st, there was no mention of him. November 2nd - nothing. November 5th - nothing. I continued to read. November 14th, there was still, not one single word about my Big Boy. I mentioned the *Garden Invaders*; Rebecca Cotton making over a neglected canal-side garden, and Kim Wilde using various ferns, grasses, herbaceous plants and heathers. And the *Big Strong Boys* were back with their MDF and ingenious lighting. But no Big Boy. I read on. It was the usual stuff. Lots of rain. Leaves on the lawn. *Coronation Street*, with Noris getting up to more mischief. Cats going to the vet. Ben gets a cold. I get Ben's cold. I start to watch *House Doctors* and *Changing Rooms*, with the lovely Laurence Llewelyn-Bowen and his floppy hair. I read all about Wendy of Weekly Wife's wonderful winter fashions, and beauty tips to fit the bill; like No 17 Plump Up The Volume lip-gloss, in Peach, and Lancôme Juicy Tube lip-gloss, in Lychee. But there was no mention of tomatoes. Big Boy must have died. I closed my diary sadly, I didn't want to read it any more. I wished I'd never started reading it again.

BUT, as I picked the diary up to put it away, an envelope fell out of the pages. It looked empty, I'd probably used it like a book mark. I was going to slip it back between the pages of the diary, then something told me to open it. And I'm glad I did. There were two photos inside. Big Boy would have had eight more tomatoes on his vine. There, in the first photo, I counted seven green tomatoes (some orangy-green) sitting happily on the kitchen work top. In the second photo, I was holding an enormous pale orange tomato, grinning like a pumpkin (I was grinning, not the tomato). I'm sure Big Boy would have been happy too, because I'd picked all his fruits. I wondered if we'd had fried green tomatoes (like in that film about a Whistle Stop café).

December

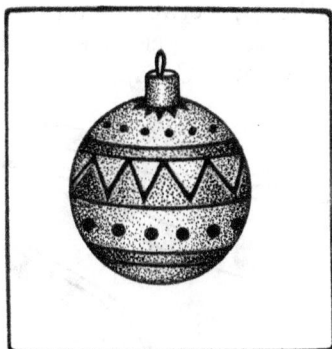

A colourful Christmas bauble greeted me in today's Advent calendar window, reminding me of the baubles on the family Christmas tree, when I was little. The chocolate snowman melted like the snowflakes on my woolly gloves, as I brushed snow off the bird table before breakfast, so the wildlife could have their breakfast. I hoped children would build another snowman in the car park.

A few more Christmas cards arrived, fluttering through the letter box with the boring post, and I had an enjoyable opening session. Among the jolly Santas, robins and mistletoe, were two more cards with meerkats wearing Santa hats. There seems to be endless TV adverts featuring humorous meerkats at the moment. And our local garden centre was full of meerkat garden ornaments, back in October. Meerkat bird baths, meerkat bird feeders, fountains and solar lights, a family of meerkats for your lawn. Meerkat mania is upon us.

I half watched the film; *Crazy for Christmas*, as I wrote the last of the Christmas cards. Then sighed with relief, as I placed a neat little pile of envelopes on the coffee table; all stamped, addressed and ready for posting on Saturday.

Curling up on the sofa like a meerkat with Mary, I browsed through a Christmas gift catalogue. The Musical Notes wall art and Diva jewellery stand caught my eye, and after dinner I showed them to Ben.

ME: What do you think of this wall art? The catalogue says; like a melody floating on a breeze, this intriguing art work captures the free unfettered spirit of music itself.

Bridging the gap between sculpture and graphic design, it's hand crafted in recycled metal and features an unknown theme in the key of C major.

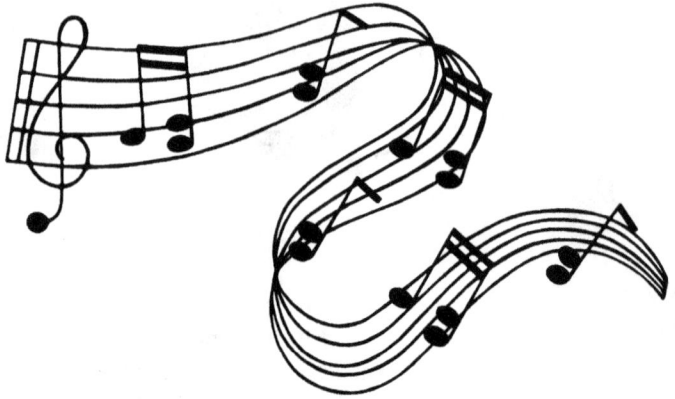

BEN: Marvellous.

ME: Yes! It would compliment our musical notes coat hooks, and violin playing cat tea-light holder.

BEN: And musical chairs.

ME: Musical chairs?

BEN: Just kidding.

ME: I never liked musical chairs as a kid.

BEN: Neither did I.

ME: I forgot to mention the musical cats, playing in a jazz band, key holder. The wall art would look wonderful on the same wall.

BEN: Anything you say dear.

ME: I like this black metal jewellery stand too.

BEN: She's got flowers sprouting out of her shoulders.

ME: Why not! Maybe it's an intriguing artwork about blossoming youth, or something. Anyway, I like the design *and* the thought of flowers growing out of my shoulders.

BEN: What are you like.

ME: Maybe there's a planet where humans sprout flowers out of their bodies on their birthday, if they are named after flowers. If you name your little girl Daisy, she will sprout daisies. Rosie will sprout roses......

BEN: Poppy sprouts poppies.

ME: I used to know a girl who had a pretty little oval face, like a tulip. She liked to wear red, so I sometimes called her Little Red Tulip.

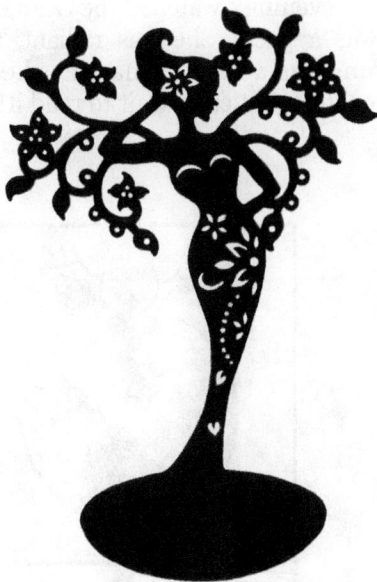

BEN: Did she mind?

ME: It made her laugh, and she would call me Verity Red Rose, if I blushed.

BEN: Did you laugh?

ME: Oh yes! I cackled.

BEN: Ivy would be a good name for you, because you love your ivy plants.

ME: Friends of the witch in my witchy book sometimes called her Ivy, because she had so many ivy plants. I could have had a storyline where she does a spell to sprout ivy out of her head.

BEN: But the book is done now.

ME: Done and printed. *Completely completed.*

* * * * * * *

Late evening I watched the Graham Norton show because Dawn French was a guest. She was radiant, like a *dawn* fresh pink rosebud. And funny as a *French* man, as she talked in an animated way about her new book. I can't wait to read it!

Saturday 18th

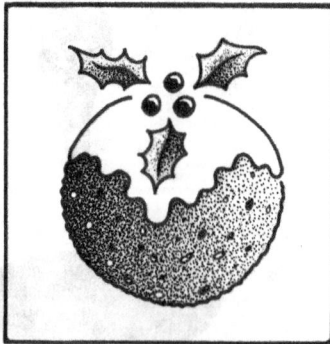

December

Ben came home from town today with a jolly Santa smile on his face. He plodded in through the front door, laden with multi-coloured carrier bags, full of Christmassy gifts and Christmassy food. Snowflakes were melting on his jacket, like today's Advent chocolate candle melted on my tongue. The Advent picture looked very tasty too, a Christmas pudding with holly on top.

ME: I see you got me lots of points on my Boots card, thanks. I also see that you were served by a Noella. I wonder if she was born on Christmas day.

BEN: Yeah.

ME: If I had a boy on Christmas day, I'd call him Rudolf.

BEN: I'm sure you would dear, especially if he had a little red nose.

ME: And if he had a twin sister I'd call her Holly.

BEN: Then you'd change your name to Ivy.

ME: Hahaha! I could sing her to sleep with *The Holly and The Ivy*, and when she was old enough to speak she'd say...

BEN: What are you like mum.

* * * * * * *

Late afternoon, I enjoyed watching little girls and boys building a snowman, and having snowball fights in the car park. Then I picked up two Christmas cards with kittens on and showed them to Ben.

ME: Now I have snowdrops on roses and whiskers on kittens.

BEN: All you need now is bright copper kettles and warm woollen mittens.

ME: I'm not too bothered about the bright copper kettles and warm woollen mittens.

BEN: In that case I'll give you brown paper packages tied up with string.

ME: Lovely!

Sunday 19th

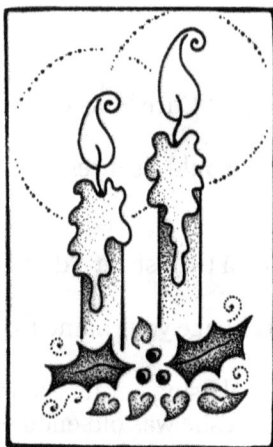

     I couldn't see the little number 19 on my Advent calendar today. Ben found it for me. The window opened to reveal festive candles, and Ben said the chocolate Christmas tree melted on his tongue like a chocolate Christmas tree.

ME: I would like a chocolate Christmas tree, a life size one, decorated with chocolate decorations.

BEN: Why does that not surprise me dear.

     I found a snail's shell in the vegetable rack at lunchtime, that did surprise me! Until I noticed on closer inspection, it was a dried up chestnut left over from last Christmas. I showed it to Ben.

Me: Look what I found in the veg rack.

BEN: Oh, that old chestnut!

ME: It has turned dark brown, the same colour as Swiss plain chocolate, made from premium grade cocoa beans, from South America and Africa.

BEN: Is that so dear.

I burst into song (well, better than bursting into tears) like you do when you find a chestnut in your vegetable rack at Christmas time, even if it is all shrivelled up and the colour of Swiss plain chocolate.

ME: *Chestnuts roasting on an open fire*
           Jack Frost nipping at your nose
           La, la la la, la la la, la la la

BEN: *Merry Christmas tooo yooo!*

Later in the day, as I watched the birds feeding in our winter wonderland, I burst into song (well, better than a burst water pipe).

ME: *Sleigh bells ring, are you listening*
           In the lane snow is glistening
           A beautiful sight, we're happy tonight

BEN: *Walking in a winter wonderland!*

Early evening, I burst into song again in the bath (better than bursting into flames) although I'm not sure the neighbours would agree.

ME: *Oh, the weather outside is frightful*
           But the fire is so delightful
           And since we've no place to go

BEN: *Let it snow! Let it snow! Let it snow!*

Monday 20th

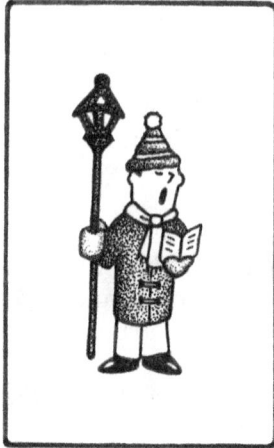

      The snow was crispy and crunchy as Kettle crisps, as I ventured into Mother Nature's freezer, first thing. After filling the bird table and bird feeders, I stood for a while, breathing in fresh freezing air..... breathing out fresh white clouds...... and feeling Jack Frost run his fingers through my hair. Bobby robin fluttered onto the fence. I felt poetic and couldn't resist quoting some verse to him, by William Wordsworth.

ME: *Art thou the bird whom man loves best, the pious bird with scarlet breast. Our little English robin, the bird that comes about our doors.*

BOBBY: What are you like (robin language).

      I couldn't remember the last part of the verse. Something about autumn winds sobbing. Or bobbing. Or something. But I felt a little inspired, as I breathed in winter and breathed out some verse.

      Jack Frost
      I know you're there
      You run your fingers
      Through my hair

December

> With an air
> Of fresh and freezy
> Your breath all white
> And breezy

ME: What do you think Jack Frost?

JACK: What are you like (Icelandic).

On my way back indoors I noticed seven bottles of Black Sheep ale, standing to attention on the window ledge. Our small fridge and tiny kitchen is so well stocked with Christmas treats, Ben must have decided to use Mother Nature's fridge to keep his ale nicely chilled.

I thought this was an excellent idea, and although the bottles looked amusing standing in a row on our snowy window ledge, I decided that black sheep would prefer to be in a field. I carefully placed the bottles in my herb patch nearby, with seven garden ornaments. Only their heads and shoulders were visible above the deep blanket of snow. Did I see Grumpy smile? Did I see Dopey's eyes light up? Did I see Doc rummage in his sack for a bottle opener? Did Happy look even happier? Did Sleepy wake up? Did Sneezy stop sneezing? Did Bashful grin?

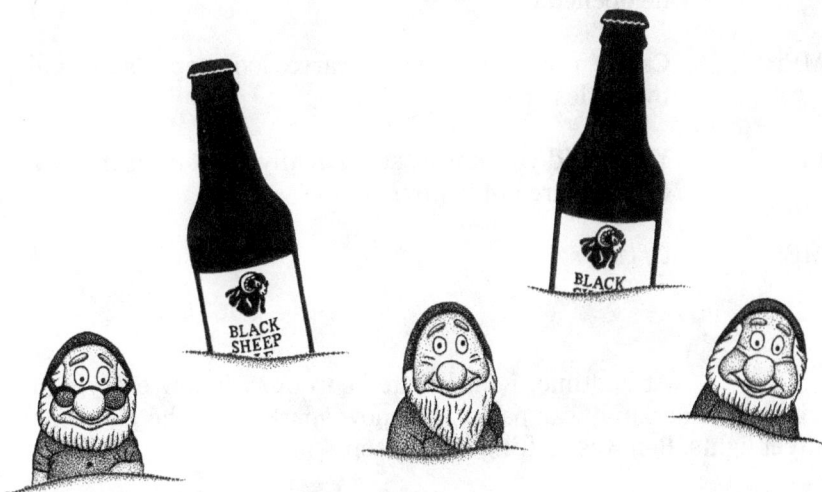

I watched shivering strangers (their shoulders hunched) crunch their way to work through the snow. Then I crunched wholemeal toast in the warmth of my kitchen (with a hunch that there would be more snow soon) watching Bobby the robin, the blue tits and goldfinches feeding outside. They looked like tiny feathery brush strokes of bright colour on Mother Nature's large snowy-white canvas. I imagined her standing and admiring her painting, head on one side, knowing she had created a perfect Christmas card scene.

There was a carol singer in today's Advent calendar window, and the chocolate reindeer melted on my tongue, like snowflakes on a warm carol singers nose. More Christmas cards arrived, some with delightful wildlife pictures: a badger in the snow, cat on a fence in the snow, and a robin nibbling Christmas cake.

When Ben came home from work, I opened the back door and shone a torch on my herb patch, so he could see his black sheep in their snowy field. He laughed.

BEN: Hey, they look cool!

ME: Yes, hahaha!

BEN: Here's a joke for you. I've just bought a friend of mine a new fridge, you should have seen his face light up when he opened it.

ME: Cackle, cackle! The seven dwarves look happy surrounded by bottles of ale, don't they.

BEN: Yeah. Did you know, statistically, six out of the seven dwarves are not happy?

ME: *Of course!*

* * * * * * *

At bedtime, I sat by the bedroom window enjoying the winter-wonderlandy car park. The snow sparkled in the glow of the street lights. Ben was drifting off to sleep.

ME: The snow looks so...... sigh...... clean and pure...... crispy and white, like a fresh clean Irish linen table cloth draped over an old wooden table.

BEN: Y..... a..... w..... n.

ME: I miss Ireland, it's too long since I visited the Emerald Isle.

BE: *Y........ A........ W........ N.*

ME: It wouldn't be the same if snow were green.... or blue.... although candy-floss pink would be nice...... hmm..... or lilac........... black would be very depressing.

BEN: Yes *dearzzzzzzzz*.

Tuesday 21ˢᵗ

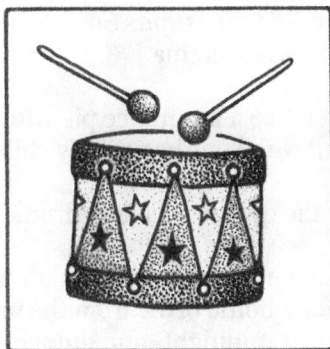

More snowflakes fell during the early hours, but today they began to melt away. The leaves on the privet hedge were dripping as I scrunched my way to the bird table. Small clumps of snow flumped to the ground. Flumped? Yes, I like that word. Or maybe shlumped is a better word. No. I like flumped.

Nutty the squirrel was passing by on the fence, so I asked his opinion.

ME: Hi Nutty, do small clumps of snow flump, or shlump to the ground?

NUTTY: What are you like (squirrel language).

   The chocolate bauble in my calendar window melted in my mouth like the snow on the privet hedge. The little picture was a drum with drum sticks, so of course I felt inspired to burst into song about twelve drummers drumming, ending with a squirrel in a sycamore tree.
   Ben returned home just after 11p.m. from his Avocado Pair gig at the Mexxa Mexxa, looking tired but happy, in a tired-but-happy-musician way.

BEN: All the Christmas tunes went down well with the diners tonight.

ME: That's great! Did *Jingle Bells* go down well with the Jalapeño poppers?

BEN: Yeah, and *The Christmas Song* went down well with the Championes con crema.

ME: Would you like a hot mince pie with brandy butter, to go down well with your beautifully chilled Black Sheep ale?

BEN: Great! If the dwarves haven't drunk it all.

   The full moon shone down spookily on the seven dwarves, as I ventured outside for a bottle of ale from the herb patch. I imagined them all coming to life at midnight, and enjoying a Christmas party, and was tempted to put out a plate of mince pies.
   While Ben washed down hot mince pies with cold ale, I asked him a question. A *very important* question. I wanted an honest opinion. A *very honest* opinion.

Me: Do clumps of snow flump or shlump when they fall to the ground?

BEN: Flump.

Wednesday 22nd

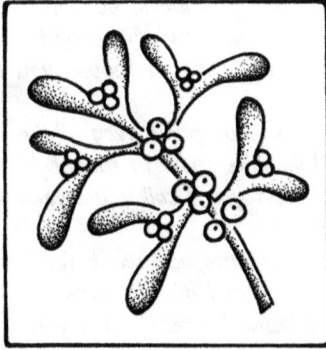

When I fed the wildlife I noticed that much of the snow had melted in my herb patch, and a couple of bottles of Black Sheep ale had fallen over. Happy and Sleepy had fallen over too. I guessed the dwarves had enjoyed their Christmas party!

Today's Advent calendar window opened to reveal a sprig of mistletoe. The chocolate holly melted on my tongue like the brandy butter on last night's mince pies, and I fancied a cold mince pie with my mid-morning mug of de-caf coffee. As I sipped, I stared out of the sitting room window and noticed (now that the trees were bare) I could see a church spire in the distance. Did this in*spire* me to write heavenly poetry? No. Did I feel Christmassy verse coming on? No. Did I feel the need to burst into song about a silent night, a holy night, a little town of Bethlehem, or a manger? No.

Cleopatra sat on my mobile phone and made the ring tone go off. This startled her, and made her pass wind. It never fails to surprise me how such a small pretty creature can make such a *big stinky* smell. Did I feel inspired? Yes, of course I did! *Everything* my cats do inspires me. I wrote a little song to the tune of Elvis Presley's hit single, *Are You Lonesome Tonight.*

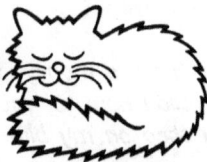

CLEOPATRA

*Are you lovely tonight
Are you cuddly tonight
When you sit on my mobile you fart*

*Are your paws very white
Like the snow in moonlight
When I kiss you I call you sweetheart*

*All the time you want feeding
But I do not care
I know I'd really miss you
If you were not there*

*With your round lovely tum
And your big hairy bum
Tell me puss
Are you lovely tonight*

* * * * * *

When Ben came home from work, he was busy chatting on his mobile phone for a while. I waited until he'd finished his last call, handed him a bottle of ale, then entertained him with my latest song in my best Elvis Presley voice. He smiled wearily, then told me a joke.

BEN: I've been on the phone for ages trying to book tickets for an Elvis tribute act, but it keeps asking me to press one for the money, two for the show.....

When I had finished cackling I picked up a box of *GoCat* crunchies, gave it a little shake-rattle-n-roll, then burst into song once more. I sang Elvis's song, *Blue Suede Shoes*, with a small change to the lyrics.

ME: *Well it's a one for the money, two for the show
Three to get ready now go, cat, go
But don't you step on my blue suede paws*

Well, you can do anything but stay off of
My blue suede paws

Ben picked up his guitar and joined in, singing with his
best Elvis impersonation. He was really good! The cats woke up, yawned,
and gave us their best *what-are-you-two-like* expressions.

BEN: *Well, you can knock me down*
          Step on my face
          Slander my name
          All over the place
          Well do anything that you want to do
          But uh~uh honey, lay off of my paws

ME: *And don't you*
          Step on my blue suede paws
          Well, you can do anything
          But lay off of my blue suede paws

Thursday 23rd

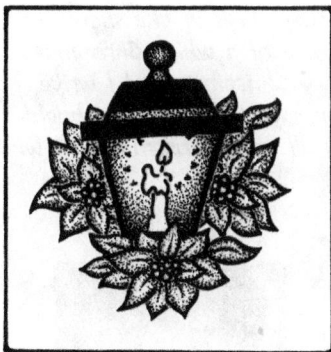

I found Sleepy lying on his back next to Dopey in the
herb patch today. Did I hear a tiny snore? Grumpy and Bashful were
leaning to one side. Did they look a little cross-eyed? I imagined another
good night had been had by all. An icy-cold wind whipped my hair
across my face as I filled the bird table. There wasn't much snow left,
but I hoped there would be some on the hills surrounding our valley

on Christmas day, so I could enjoy the sight on our way to my sister's house in Gillingham. I've always dreamed of a white Christmas, just like Bing Crosby in his 1942 rendition of *White Christmas*, written by Burl Ives. The best selling single of all time.

    After I opened my Advent calender window (a lamp with poinsettia) I opened a couple of Christmas cards, and both were very beautiful religious paintings; *Madonna with baby Jesus* by Carlo Maratta (1625-1713) and *Madonna and child* by Giovanni Battista Salvi (1609-85). I studied them for a while, enjoying the amazing use of colour and light; and felt inspired to draw a pencil sketch of Mary (my little cat, not the Virgin Mary).

    Today's chocolate reindeer melted on my tongue, like my heart melted when I saw the reindeer on the Trevarno Estate website.

2.20p.m.   I sang in the bath, under a quilt of frothy snowy-white bubbles.

> *I'm dreaming of a white Christmas*
> *Just like the ones I used to know*
> *Where the tree tops glisten*
> *And children listen*
> *To hear sleigh bells in the snow*
> *I'm dreaming of a white Christmas*
> *With every Christmas card I write*
> *May your days be merry and bright*
> *And may all your Christmases be white*

Friday 24th

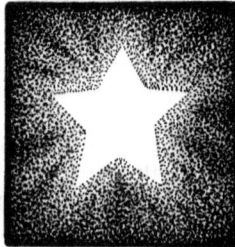

    A gold star (on a Cadbury's purple background) greeted me today when I opened the last Advent calendar window; the chocolate

Santa melting on my tongue, like my heart when I opened today's Christmas card. The picture on the front was a Victorian painting of Santa with a sack full of toys. Inside my friend Len had written a delightful poem.

> *A wizard lived on Buckland Hill*
> *For all we know, he lives there still*
> *He wrote poems of this and that*
> *Of furry moggies thin and fat*
> *But when it comes to Christmas time*
> *He stuck to only one good rhyme*
> *The important thing he would say*
> *Was to wish you well on Christmas day*

9.00 a.m.   After I'd given the bird's their festive treat (Bill Oddie's Premium Really Wild bird food - cereals for slow-release energy, oil rich sunflower seeds and tiny seeds for small birds - with no funny coloured pellets or cheap fillers you might find in other mixes), I put lots of peanuts out for the squirrels. Then I treated myself to a hot (a bit too hot) mince pie for breakfast, while I watched the animation of Charles Dickens's novel set in Victorian London, *A Christmas Carol*.

11.00 a.m.   I dozed on the sofa with the hairy children, watching *The Muppet's Christmas Carol*. I do love Kermit and Miss Piggy. Michael Caine too.

12.30 p.m.   Ben sent me a text:

THREE WISE WOMEN WOULD HAVE ASKED DIRECTIONS, ARRIVED ON TIME, BROUGHT PRACTICAL GIFTS, CLEANED THE STABLE, MADE A CASSEROLE, AND THERE WOULD BE PEACE ON EARTH - BX

12.31 p.m.   I replied:

HEHEHE, WOT DO U GET WEN U CROSS A SNOWMAN WITH A VAMPIRE ?

12.32 p.m. Ben replied:

DUNNO, WOT DO U GET WEN U CROSS A SNOWMAN WITH A VAMPIRE ?

12.32 p.m. FROST BITE

12.33 p.m. HAHAHA - POPPIN INTO SAINS-B ON WAY HOME - ANYTHIN YOU WANT TO ADD TO LIST ?

12.35 p.m. ERM - OOH - UMM - AHHH - MORE CRACKERS AND PICKLES - TO GO WITH THE CHEEZ PLEEZ

12.37 p.m. OK - AND BY THE WAY - WOT DO HEDGEHOGS EAT FOR LUNCH ?

12.38 p.m. DUNNO - WOT DO HEDGEHOGS EAT FOR LUNCH ?

12.39 p.m. PRICKLED ONIONS

12.40 p.m. HEHEHE - WE ARE IN JOLLY FESTIVE SPIRITS

12.42 p.m. DO WE NEED ANY SPIRITS ?

12.43 p.m. NO - OUR RESIDENT SPOOKS ARE QUITE ENUF - BUT I FANCY SUMTHIN XMASSY AND SWEET

12.45 p.m. ME IN A SANTA SUIT ?

12.46 p.m. HAHAHA

12.48 p.m. WUD YOU LIKE SUM OF THOSE ROUND CHOCS WRAPPED IN GOLD ? YOU CALL THEM FURRY ROCHETS

12.50 p.m. OOH - OK - IF U INSIST X

3.05 p.m. Ben came home with Sainsbury's carrier bags, a Santa smile and a sackful of goodies. Well not exactly a sack, more a large red carrier bag. He is a buyer for a fire alarms company, and every Christmas his suppliers give him gifts; usually port, wine, whisky or a Christmas pudding. This year he brought home wine, port, and an enormous wedge of cheese. When he gave me the cheese to put in the fridge, I noticed it had an unusual name.

ME: Grand piano cheese? Is it the colour of piano keys?

BEN: You have your M.E. eyeballs in today dear.

ME: Oh, it's Grand Padano cheese!

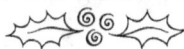

6.45 p.m.   Nibbling grand piano with pickle on a crackers, I watched, *Scrooge: A Christmas Carol*. The vintage 1951 adaptation of Charles Dickens's novel. I think I prefer the 1992 adaptation, *The Muppet's Christmas Carol*.

Saturday 25th

7.35 a.m   Ben finds the lumpy sock full of treats, Santa has left for him at the end of the bed.

7.37 a.m.   There's a lot of rustling and munching.

ME: Happy Cadbury's Christmas Ben!

7.45 a.m.   The cats sniff at their Christmas stocking, full of fishy treats and toys.

7.46 a.m.   There's a lot of crunching and jingling sounds.

ME: Happy festive fun my three hairy children!

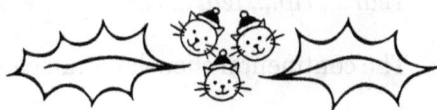

8.01 a.m.	I put out more of Bill Oddie's luxury wild bird food, and piles of peanuts for the wildlife.
8.02 a.m.	I notice Ben has put empty bottles of Black Sheep ale back in the herb patch for a joke. Sleepy is lying on his back next to Dopey and Happy. Grumpy, Bashful and Sneezy, are leaning against the empty bottles. Doc has fallen over on his side.
ME:	A very Merry Christmas my seven dwarves!
8.03 a.m.	As soon as I step indoors the wildlife appear. There's a lot of wild pecking and nibbling.
ME:	Happy festive feeding, birds and squirrels!
8.15 a.m.	I crunch my toast, then treat myself to a Hazelnut praline and Almond crunch.
ME:	A very crunchy Christmas to me!
8.27 a.m.	Text message from Jayne:
	THANK YOU SO MUCH – I LOVE THE SLIPPER SOCKS – I NEEDED NEW ONES SO THEY ARE PERFECT – XMASSY HUGS XXX
8.30 a.m.	I reply:
	MERRY XMAS WITCHY FRIEND – LOVED YOR KITTEN XMAS CARD – WARM FESTIVE HUGS XXX
8.45 a.m.	*Tear..... rip... rip... tear.... rustle.*
BEN:	Cheers for the cool continental shirt, it's great!
	Tear.... rip.... tear....rip.
ME:	The continental chocolates are cool too!

Rip... rustle...rip...rustle.

BEN: Mmm, these chilli treats look very tasty. Seriously hot mustard.... Caribbean hot sauce.... chilli jam.... delicious!

ME: The chocs are very tasty too, and I love the pink baby-sleep-suit for grown-ups.

Tear.... tear.... rustle.... rip.... tear.

BEN: Thanks for the car stuff Santa.

Rip... rip... rip...rustle... rip.

ME: Thanks for the bath stuff Santa.

Tear.... rip.... rustle.... rip.... rustle.

BEN: 'I LOVE DADDY' socks, thanks cats!

Rip.... tear.... rustle.... rustle.

ME: Oh! this is a sweet little silver trinket box, I like the tiny mouse on top, thanks cats!

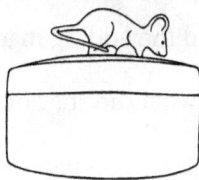

BEN: I forgot I'd bought this for you until this morning and we've run out of Christmassy wrapping paper, so here you are, a *very merry Bill Bailey* Christmas dear.

ME: *Dandelion Mind!* Great, I'd completely forgotten I wanted this DVD.

10.00 a.m.	*Tap... tap... tap.* Ben is sitting at his computer, sending seasons greetings to family and friends abroad and in the West Country. *Splish... splash... splish.* I'm in the bath enjoying my new Lush soap and bath fizzer from Santa, and hoping Dawn French is having a good Christmas in the West Country. I expect it will be a happy one if she has sold lots of copies of her new book. I'm sure she will have, she's promoted it so well. I hope my sister managed to buy me a copy, even though I didn't get the title *exactly* right when I texted her.
11.00 a.m.	*Chop.... chop... chop.* Ben is preparing a vegetarian Christmas for two. Wonderful!
11.25 a.m.	*Clink.... clink.... clink.* I lay the Christmas table with shiny cutlery and glasses, red and gold serviettes, a red candle in a festive holder, and shiny gold crackers.
1.15 p.m.	*Crack! Crack!* We pull the gold crackers. *Rustle, Rustle.* We don gold paper hats.
1.17 p.m.	*Rattle! Rattle!* We wind up the plastic toy gifts. Ben's owl chases my mouse across the table.
1.19 p.m.	We read out the jokes.
BEN:	What did the adding machine say to the clerk?
ME:	Dunno, what did the adding machine say to the clerk?
BEN:	You can count on me.
ME:	What did the plate say to the other plate?
BEN:	Umm, dunno, what did the plate say to the other plate?
ME:	Lunch is on me.

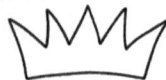

1.25 p.m.	We enjoy a delicious Christmas dinner; home-made nut roast, with roast potatoes, sprouts, parsnips, chestnuts and gravy.
3.00 p.m.	Dozing in front of Christmas TV, paper hats askew.
4.35 p.m.	Jackets and boots on, laden with bags of gifts, we climb into the car.
5.05 p.m.	MERRY CHRISTMAS EVERYONE !
5.10 p.m.	We exchange presents round the Christmas tree. Lots of rips, rustling and thankyous.
5.12 p.m.	*Hurrah!* My sister has given me Dawn French's new book, *A Tiny Bit Marvellous*. I have a quick peek at a few pages; and like a big box of beautifully inviting chocolates, I can't resist dipping into it for a couple of tasty *tiny-bit-marvellous* treats.

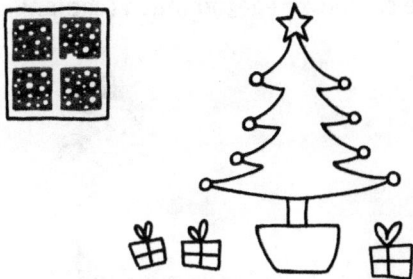

I'm going to really enjoy slowly devouring the whole book over the festive period (when I can keep awake). Every chapter will be a delightfully different delicious flavour. And one day, when I live next to Dawn, I will pop round to see her, and tell her about all the parts I loved best. Maybe I'll give her a copy of my *tiny-bit-witchy* book. We'll chat for ages about writing (eating chocolates) and I'll imagine I'm a famous celebrity writer too, with my picture on the cover of Weekly Wife. And we'll laugh a lot.

6.00.p.m.	Time for the Time Lord, in the Christmas episode of *Doctor Who*. Amy and the doctor encounter a scrooge-like-miser in, *A Christmas Carol*. My sister, niece and nephew, their dog and I, get comfortable on the floor of their *tiny-but-marvellous* sitting room. Ben, my brother, brother-in-law, his brother and my dad, doze on the three piece suite. All eyes on the *rather-big-marvellous* TV screen.
7.00 p.m.	Time for tea, with tasty home-made Christmas cake on festive paper plates.
10.00 p.m.	Time to go home.
11.00 p.m.	Time for bed.
ME:	That was a marvellous Christmas day.... *Y.... A....W.... N.*
BEN:	Yeah.... *Y..... A.....W..... N......* Burp.. I've eaten too much.
CATS:	Purrrrrrrrrrrrrr. *Y... A... A... W... W... N. Purrrrrrrrrrrrr.* We can never eat too much (cat language).

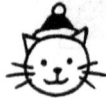

Sunday 26th

I awoke to a winter wonderland. Jack Frost had been very busy, even snowmen would be shivering. The garden was so white I thought it had snowed over night. Wishful thinking.

Though I felt extremely exhausted after yesterday, I couldn't resist singing quietly to myself as I put the kettle on for Boxing Day breakfast. I fancied a mince pie instead of toast.

ME:	*Sleigh bells ring, are you listening* *In the lane, snow is glistening*
BEN:	*A beautiful sight, we're happy tonight*

ME: *Walking in a winter wonderland.......Yawn.*

BEN: You look exhausted, I'll feed the cats and birds.

ME: Thanks..... *Yawn.......* Sneeze.

      I wore my pink baby-sleep-suit, with zebra print arms. Its warmth and cotton-wool-softness was most comforting, and the little embroidered zebra motif made me smile. I curled up on the sofa with my cats, like a contented pink baby cuddling her toys. There was a lot of purring and dozing, and the occasional snore (feline and human). I turned on the TV with the volume low. Cleopatra wanted to watch *Carry on Cleo,* so we watched that, followed by *Carry on Henry* and *Carry on Camping.*

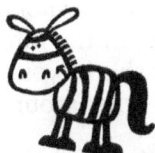

      After dinner I read a little of, *A Tiny Bit Marvellous,* savouring every delicious paragraph. Dawn French's crazy humour made me laugh so much, I almost wet myself (well, I think I did, a tiny bit). But that was OK, because you are allowed to wet yourself when you are a big baby.
      When I needed to go to the bathroom, I crawled on my hands and knees across the sitting room floor to make Ben laugh. I was so tired, I really *did* have to crawl on my hands and knees, up the mountain of stairs to the bathroom.
      Late evening we watched the film, *Love Actually.* I laughed a lot. I cried a lot. Babies are expected to cry a lot, so I happily dipped into the Kleenex, from the *very* beginning to the *very* end of the film. But I really enjoyed myself. Actually. Then after a milky drink, I crawled slowly up to bed to sleep peacefully. Like a baby.

Monday 27th

      I found the energy to wallow in a bath late afternoon, and poured lots of Happy Hippo bubble bath under the hot running tap. As

I daydreamed under mountains of frothy bubbles, Ben wandered into the bathroom.

ME: I'd like a yellow plastic duck to play with in the bath, now that I'm a big pink baby.

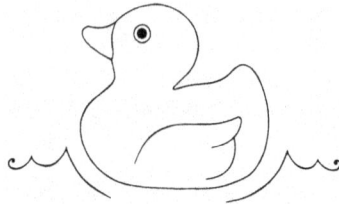

BEN: Of course dear, babies should have a yellow plastic duck, I'll find you one on the internet. You can play with the wind-up plastic sharks you gave me last year if you like, they chase each other around the bath.

ME: That sounds fun!

* * * * * *

After a playful bath (the most fun I've ever had at bathtime, apart from when I put my collection of resin sea creatures into the water and pretended to be swimming in the sea) I climbed into my cosy warm baby-sleep-suit to watch, *Three Men and a Baby* with Mary. Ben laughed when he saw the film I was watching, and heard me sing along as the men serenaded the baby to sleep.

ME: *Goodnight sweetheart, well it's time to go*
      Goodnight sweetheart, well it's time to go
      I hate to leave you but I really must say
      Goodnight sweetheart, goodnight.

BEN: Would you like me to sing you to sleep with that song dear?

ME: Oh yes (hahaha) you could work out some chords for the chorus!

295

BEN: Certainly dear.

ME: I love Ted Dansen, he was brilliant in *Cheers* and *Loch Ness*. Love Tom Selleck too. I read in Weekly wife that he got quite broody making the film, what a sweetheart.

BEN: Yes dear.

ME: I don't know the other chap, on the right, do you?

BEN: It'll probli be in the TV mag (rustle rustle rustle) which channel?

ME: Four.

BEN: Ah, Steve Guttenburg.

ME: Oh, never heardovim, but he's good too.

Tuesday 28th

Rain washed away the last traces of snow during the night. The garden looked gloomy. Stale chocolate browns. Sad slimy greens. Old boot browns. Mouldy greens. Sluggish browns. No more white in sight.

To brighten my sluggish and mouldy-greeny-old-boot-brown mood, I wrapped a colourful shawl around my dressing gown. The dazzling oranges, sunshine yellows, glowing greens and Christmassy crimsons worked a treat. The long delicate tassels fluttered, as braved the freezing cold wind on my way to feed the wildlife.

I curled up with Dawn French after lunch. Well, not exactly the woman herself (although I imagine she's nice and cuddly) more her wonderful sense of humour. I had read as far as the third page of chapter twelve, page 36, when I *almost* wet myself again (laughing out loud) as I read the conversation between Mo and her teenage daughter. It's one of those books that's very hard to put down, even when your eyes start to close like a sleepy baby.

I closed my eyes. Then I heard Ben softly singing, '*Goodnight sweetheart, well it's time to go*'. I giggled, then eventually nodded off, cuddling the book resting open on my chest. When I awoke I noticed Ben had left a Cadbury's Flake wrapper on the coffee table, and decided to use it as a bookmark, shaking a few choccy crumbs into my mouth first (I knew Dawn would approve, as I recalled her in the Terry's chocolate orange advert). Ben decided to bleed the radiators, and while he did this, I curled up with Purrdita to watch the comedy film, *Baby's Day Out.*

BEN: There's going to be a lot of loud gurgling from the radiators in a minute.

ME: There's going to be a lot of loud gurgling and baby laughter from the TV in a minute.

Wednesday 29th

Today was Ben's family-Christmas-get-together at his sister's house. I'm always too tired and fatigued to make the long journey and be sociable, after my sister's family-Christmas-get-together. I'm like the garden when the rain has washed away the last of the snow; there's no more sparkle. No more white. My snowman has left me to visit his family. I'm dull. Dull. Dull. Dull. My mood is mouldy and muddy. My thoughts sluggish. I'm stale as old chocolate. I'm sad-slimy-green and old-boot-brown. Downtrodden. Flat. A Christmas Cinderella, sitting by the fireside. Grey as ashes. Completely burnt out. Home alone. All by myself. And I don't feel like bursting into song about being *all by myself,* like Bridget Jones wearing her pyjamas and pretending to play a drum kit.

BUT THIS YEAR! This year, I felt happy, wearing my fluffy and cosy-cotton-wooly-baby-sleep-suit. So *very* soft. So *very* marshmallowy-pink. I was toasty warm and comforted. And it didn't matter that I was putting on weight, because there's lots of room in a sleep-suit, and it's compulsory for babies to put on weight. *And* we still had a fridge full of tasty naughty-but-nice treats, and babies can be naughty-but-nice. AND I had Dawn French and my cats to cuddle up with.

There were some good films on TV, like *The Holiday* (with the handsome what's-his-name, Kate Winslet, and Cameron Diaz) and *The Very Merry Christmas Muppet Movie* (with the lovely Kermit and Miss Piggy). *AND* it had been a great year because I had managed to complete my witchy book, *Love & Best Witches.* It was *finally* done, beautifully printed, well received, *and* A.F.M.E. had given me a double-page spread in InterAction, *all to myself.* So it didn't matter *at all* this year, that I was all by myself. I was contented. Pink, fluffy and smiling.

After reading a chapter of Dawn's book (which wasn't too tiring because her chapters are short, and her writing style is easy to read) I watched the film, *Death Becomes Her.* I love Goldie Hawn and Meryl Streep. Bruce Willis was great too, but not half as lovely, *nowhere near as lovely,* as the delicious Death By Chocolate cheesecake I enjoyed after dinner. It was a small dinner, just a slice of quiche and salad, because I needed lots of room in my baby tummy for a large slice of cheesecake. I liked the spooky writing on the cheesecake box; a devil's fork on the **D**, horns and pointy tail on the **C**. It made me cackle like a baby witch.

Death by Chocolate

7.30 p.m.   It's not a good idea to eat dark chocolate, especially *very dark* Death by Chocolate cheesecake; when you are tired and wearing a marshmallow pink sleep-suit, and you have M.E. so your hand-eye co-ordination isn't always that good.

8.30 p.m.   It's not a good idea to sip a glass of mulled red wine (with cinnamon and herbs) full to the brim, or bite into a Bailey's chocolate liqueur (delicious gift from dad) when you are wearing pale pink and your mind and body is *so very sleepy.*

Thursday 30th

Ben drove to Sainsbury's today to purchase crackers (to go with the tasty looking pickles and cheeses from his family), bread, and brandy butter, to go with the last of the Christmas pudding. He also nipped into town to buy me some thank you notelets, button cell batteries and guitar strings for himself.

ME: Thanks for getting the notelets, the jungle pictures are sweet and the zebra matches the zebra on my baby-sleep-suit.

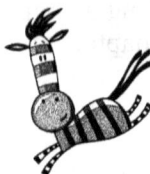

BEN: That's wonderful dear. You're not wearing it today?

ME: It's in the washing machine, I got chocolate and wine down the front.

BEN: You babies are so mucky.

ME: It's allowed, you expect babies to get grubby.

BEN: Yes dear.

ME: These Energiser button cell batteries look like little silver tablets! I'll just pop one in my mouth to energise me for the whole of 2011.

BEN: What are you like.

ME: I'm like a big baby, we put anything in our mouth.

BEN: Yeah, I know. I see you've been enjoying the Death by Chocolate cheesecake.

ME: Mmm, it went down very well with that film, *Death Becomes Her*.

BEN: What's this you're watching?

ME: Oh, just some programme called *Spice Trip*. I thought it would be a nice little programme about the Spice Girls on tour, but it's a culinary travel show about cinnamon trees in India.

BEN: Never mind dear.

Friday 31ˢᵗ

After breakfast, I sat wearing my beautifully clean pink baby-sleep-suit, gazing thoughtfully at a photograph on our sitting room wall; wild geese flying, silhouetted against an orange sunset. I felt very peaceful as I sighed deeply, and wondered how another year had flown by so quickly.

ME: Another year almost over, the years *really do* fly past faster when you get older.

BEN: *Yeah!*

ME: My nephew is learning to drive. How is this possible? He was only a toddler riding on his tricycle last year! My niece is a teenager and into rock music. How is this possible? I was rocking her in her pram, only yesterday!

2.00 p.m.   We watched the film, *Bedknobs and Broomsticks,* and I sang along quietly to myself in a sleepy-witch way.

Bobbing along, bobbing along
On the bottom of the beautiful briny sea
What a chance to get a better peep
At the plants and creatures of the deep

We glide
Far below the rolling tide
Serene
Through the lovely blue and green

It's lovely bobbing along......

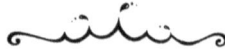

ME:　　　　I would like a magical bed like that, so I can bob along on
　　　　　the bottom of the sea and visit magical islands with talking
　　　　　animals. Everyone who has M.E. should have one, then
　　　　　we'd *never* get bored or lonely!

BEN:　　　 Yes dear, *I quite agree*, I'll look on the internet for you.

* * * * * *

　　　　Late afternoon Ben received three text messages, all the
same, from work colleagues:

　　　　BY THE SUN SETS ON 2010
　　　　BY THE MEMORIES FADE
　　　　BY THE NETWORKS GET JAMMED
　　　　BY I GET DRUNK — LOSE MY PHONE
　　　　I-M WISHING YOU A HAPPY NEW YEAR X

　　　　I felt inspired to send my own version of the message to
witchy friends:

　　　　BY THE SUN SETS ON 2010
　　　　AND THE MOON SHINES ON BAT WINGS
　　　　BY MEMORIES FADE OF SABBATS
　　　　AND SAMHAIN
　　　　BY THE NETWORKS GET JAMMED
　　　　BY I GET MERRY ON PUMPKIN WINE
　　　　AND FALL OFF MY BROOMSTICK
　　　　I-M SENDING LOVE AND BEST WITCHES
　　　　FOR A HAPPY NEW YEAR X V X

11.00 p.m.　 We settled down with the cats to watch *Jools Holland's
　　　　　Hootenany* 2010 on BBC 2.

Midnight.　 We raised our glasses of bubbly.

ME: *Happy New Year!*

BEN: *Happy New Year!*

ME: Why didn't the skeleton go to the New Year's Eve party?

BEN: Dunno, why didn't the skeleton go to the New Year's Eve party?

ME: He had no body to go with.

BEN: What has no body and no nose ?

ME: Hmm....... well, it's not Rudolf the reindeer because he has a lovely hairy reindeer body and a shiny red nose sip........ sip..... giggle....... I don't know, what has no body and no nose?

BEN: Nobody knows.

* * * * * *

12.04 a.m.   I've done it! I've done it! *Yes! Yes!!! Yes!!!!!!!!!!!!!!!!!!!* I've survived *another year!* Twelve out of *twelve!* Full marks for *me!* Another year of coping with M.E. And myself. And I'm still alive. And I'm *still* sane.
Well, most days.

12.05 a.m.   I deserve a BIG GOLD STAR. A shiny star, like you would find on the top of a Christmas tree. As big as my bedroom wall. No, *bigger.* High as the billboards in town. Tall and magnificent as the sycamore trees at the end of my garden. Tall as a tree..... I've survived M.E...... a little bit..... little bit marvellous me! Do I feel a poem coming on?........ No. Not tonight.

Maybe next year.

ME: When you are next in town, would you mind getting me a new diary?

BEN: Certainly dear.

THE END